SIMPLE GUIDE
TO USING
HOMEOPATHY

ABOUT THE AUTHOR

KEITH SMITH LCPH, MHMA, lived for a time in the picturesque village of Brightwell cum Sotwell, where Edward Bach grew and developed the famous Bach Flower Remedies in his cottage garden. As a lay herbalist Keith was unable to cure the tonsillitis from which he had suffered for twenty years. In the late 1970s he came across a small self-treatment guide to homeopathy – but was still unable to stop the recurrent tonsillitis. What the book had failed to tell him was that *chronic* tonsillitis requires the expertise of a professional homeopath.

In 1989 Keith was diagnosed as suffering from ME or Chronic Fatigue Syndrome. On his journey to recovery with the support of homeopathic treatment, he gained many hard-earned insights into how we become ill and what we need to do in order to regain our well-being.

In 1997 Keith and his wife, Linda, graduated from The Practical College of Homeopathy, West Midlands, England. Today, Keith practises in SE Kent, supporting a very wide clientele and is a highly-regarded practitioner.

This book is dedicated to his family whose support has made anything possible – and to everyone who seeks true healing.

COVER ILLUSTRATION

MINERALS and plants are two of the sources from which homeopathic tablets are prepared. This illustration includes gold (*Aurum metallicum*), silver (*Argentum metallicum*), red onion (*Allium cepa*) and ginger (*Zingiber*). The remedies are mostly given in tablet form, and may look identical to these Sulphur 6x tablets.

SIMPLE GUIDE
TO USING

HOMEOPATHY

KEITH SMITH
LCPH, MHMA

GLOBAL BOOKS LTD

Simple Guides • Series 4
NATURAL HEALTH

Simple Guide to Using
HOMEOPATHY
by Keith Smith LCPH, MHMA

First Published 2001 by

GLOBAL BOOKS LTD
PO Box 219, Folkestone, Kent, England CT20 3LZ

ISBN 1–86034–062–8

British Library Cataloguing in Publication Data
A CIP catalogue entry for this book
is available from the British Library

Set in Times New Roman 11 on 12pt by Mark Heslington, Scarborough, North Yorkshire
Printed in England by The Cromwell Press, Trowbridge, Wiltshire

Contents

Foreword
•••••

T o hear as I did, a doctor on TV say that catching meningitis or chicken-pox and suffering complications as a result, comes 'out of the blue' and is 'a lottery' is bizarre. You might expect that sort of comment from a primitive superstitious society, but a practitioner of a science-based profession? The reason that some orthodox practitioners resort to comments like these, is simply that they cannot see the process whereby one individual will catch meningitis, while another will be completely unaffected. But, to medical practitioners who take the time to find out about their patients' history and lifestyle, there is generally no mystery.

We soon learn that if the explanation is not immediately apparent we need to look a little further, not dismiss it as 'a lottery'. These sorts of comments create fear and panic, and encourage people to feel like helpless victims, whose only protection is vaccines and drugs. This is a good marketing position for the drug companies, but far from the truth.

What would be more helpful would be empowerment of the individual through the acknowledgement that we have a great degree of influence over our health, and therefore responsibility to look after ourselves. Through eating, rest, and by avoiding toxicity (both physical and emotional), we can always be healthier than if we do not look after ourselves and simply demand a quick fix from the doctor.

Fortunately, homeopathy focuses on the whole patient, which gives us very clear insights into why particular individuals get sick, even why they get a particular disease. Drawing on their own medical history and that of their family, it is even possible to ascertain their likely susceptibility to diseases in the future.

Parents have been taking their children to parties to expose them to childhood diseases for generations. This is because a healthy child will generally deal far better with these diseases than they would catching them as an adult. Much better, therefore, to get chicken pox over with as a child than to risk catching it as an adult. Children will normally be healthier when they have thrown off these childhood diseases through their own efforts. Their systems will have changed as a result of overcoming the disease, and consequently they are likely to be less susceptible in future.

However, this natural sort of immunity is very different from that claimed by vaccination. The latter involves injecting toxic materials and viruses directly into the blood stream, thus effectively bypassing the body's first lines of defence. Imagine the onslaught on the body's defences when a young baby has assorted toxins and viruses directly injected into its bloodstream even before its ability to attempt to deal with such things is fully developed. Apart from any acute reaction to the vaccine, what we see time and time again is an aggravation of former susceptibilities such as glue ear, tonsillitis, asthma, eczema etc.

No wonder some parents prefer to expose their children to childhood diseases such as german measles and chicken pox, in the knowledge that we have developed the ability over generations to deal with the virus safely as infants. In addition, our natural immune response will ensure that we do not contract german measles later on – while pregnant, for instance, when it could be harmful to the unborn baby. In contrast, more than fourteen per cent of vaccinated individuals have been found not to produce antibodies to the disease concerned. However, they could mistakenly believe that the vaccination has protected them which, self-evidently, could have serious consequences later on in life.

Should the individual for any reason struggle to deal with a natural virus, they can be treated with appropriate homeopathic remedies, in order to support them in their attempts to reject the disease.

Diseases are all around all of us continually. Our best protection is to be fit and healthy. In addition to the factors mentioned above, a wide variety of therapies are available to help us achieve and maintain an optimum level of health. Occasional constitutional homeopathic treatment can help us to achieve and retain a healthy state in the face of twenty-first century pressures such as pollution and stress. As Louise Pasteur, father of the germ theory, said shortly before he died 'disease is nothing, the soil is everything'.

We need to focus not so much on the disease, but on the soil in which disease can flourish – our minds, bodies and spirits.

The aim of this book is to encourage and support you, the reader, in the use of homeopathy, to enable you to seek the best of health for yourself and your children, to know when and how to treat yourself and your family, and when and how to seek help from a professional homeopath.

KEITH SMITH
Summer 2001

THE ORGANON
The role of the physician in sickness and in health

The physician's highest and only calling is to restore health to the sick, which is called healing.

The highest ideal of cure is rapid, gentle and permanent restoration of health . . .

He (the physician) is likewise a preserver of health if he knows the things that derange health and cause disease, and how to remove them from persons in health.

Quotations from *The Organon* by Samuel Hahnemann – the philosophy upon which homeopathy is based. It uses the principle of symptom similarity, which is the medical application of Sir Isaac Newton's Third Law of Motion: 'Action and reaction are equal and opposite'.

1 .....

The Philosophy of Homeopathic Medicine

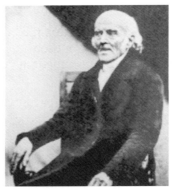

SAMUEL HAHNEMANN, 1755–1843
The creator of homeopathy

In 1796 Samuel Hahnemann, a German physician and chemist, developed a new way to heal the sick. He called this new form of medicine *homeopathy*, from the Greek words meaning 'similar suffering', and set out his philosophy in a book entitled *The Organon: The Role of the Physician in Sickness and in Health*.

Like Hippocrates in the fourth century BC, Hahnemann had realized that you could treat the sick by applying an opposite force to the sickness or a similar force. Orthodox treatment developed the system of using medicines to produce opposite effects to the patient's symptoms, which would aim to cancel out the illness. Homeopathy uses medicine which in a healthy person would produce symptoms similar to those seen in the patient to be cured. This stimulates the patient her/himself to respond against the direction of force of the medicine (and of course the symptoms), restoring a natural health.

For this reason we call orthodox medicine allopathy (opposite suffering), as opposed to homeopathy, which through same suffering, stimulates the body's own power to heal itself.

However, the great advantage of homeopathic medicine, lies in Hahnemanns' discovery that by a special process of dilution and agitation we can get rid of the potentially harmful chemical side-effects common to so many orthodox drugs, while retaining that which stimulates the curative response in the patient. Even more remarkable is that the more we dilute and agitate (or succuss) the original remedy, the greater is its potency, or capacity to produce a curative response in the patient.

☐

One of the major advantages of homeopathy is that we do not have to think we know exactly what complaint someone is suffering from before we can help them. We simply need to find a remedy that matches the symptoms that are evident in the patient. Why is this such an advantage? Simply because we can use the facts before our eyes; the first-hand evidence of the person sitting in front of us. We may be aware of the diagnosis, but we are also aware that they are very often wrong. Fortunately, we do not have to base a treatment on such an uncertain premise, nor do we have to subject a patient to batteries of unpleasant, worrying and potentially harmful tests. Instead, we are guided by careful observation of the symptoms, the constitution and the past medical history of the patient and their family.

Many people choose homeopathy as a last resort, when allopathic treatment has not only failed to produce a cure itself (as it always must), but has caused additional health problems. Sometimes these result from suppression. This is when the original symptoms (the body's attempt to cure) are stopped, forcing the sickness to a deeper and more serious level within the patient. Often, the additional health problems result from the side-effects of prescribed drugs. Complaints like vertigo, high blood pressure, Parkinson's disease, cancer etc. can all be caused by prescribed drugs and other forms of orthodox treatment, so it is no surprise that many patients eventually withdraw from the aggressive mechanistic and weakening approach of drugging, cutting, burning, freezing etc. and opt for the supportive, strengthening process of homeopathy.

Increasingly, homeopathy and other therapies are becoming the first choice for a disillusioned public.

This despite the fact that, unfortunately, it is often less accessible than they would like, due to the continuing political support for the very powerful and wealthy drug companies. The more we learn from an early age to take responsibility for our health – mental, physical and emotional, then, increasingly, in the future we will not tolerate much of what passes today for medical treatment; the suppression of the disease but at what cost to the patient's overall health?

Because homeopathic remedies are diluted to minute doses, they do not damage organs or turn people's minds or emotions off. Instead, they help the physical, mental and emotional (whole person) to process their disease and thereby reach a higher level of health. This is a true cure, rather than suppression by continually having to supply an opposing force to stop symptoms reappearing; or surgically cutting something out and hoping you can weaken the body so much with cocktails of toxic chemicals that it will not grow back. Surgery and drugs do have their uses of course, but preferably as a last resort!

Antibiotics are becoming less effective due to the development of resistant strains of bacteria and many people are reluctant to risk the side-effects of steroids. Homeopathy offers a very safe and well-proven alternative – one that does not seek to stop the body from *showing* the symptoms of ill health, but rather seeks to restore health so that the individual no longer has any reason to produce symptoms.

2
· · · · ·

Remedies and their Effects

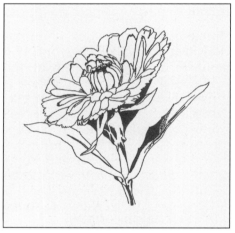

POT MARIGOLD
Source of the homeopathic remedy
calendula

H omeopathic remedies are obtained from mineral, vegetable, animal and biological materials. Through seeing the effects of using the specially prepared remedies on patients, Dr Samuel Hahnemann established the following principles:

THE HAHNEMANN PRINCIPLES

- A substance, which in a crude dose will cause a disease, will in small doses cure that disease.

- Through extreme dilution, poisonous and harmful side-effects are lost, while the healing power of the remedy is enhanced.

- Homeopathic remedies are prescribed after carefully considering all aspects of the individual's constitution, temperament and responses to disease

That remedies have profound effects on humans and animals is evident from two hundred years of use. However, exactly how they work is still not known. After all, the remedies are often so diluted, that no chemical traces of the original substance remain. Instead, the active healing properties appear to be imparted to the water in which they are diluted during preparation. Somewhat like the way in which a voice can be converted to an electro-magnetic energy pattern which can be transmitted to your receiver (telephone or radio), and be experienced as if it has the qualities of the original voice.

In this example, we know that the voice is disembodied, but the electro-magnetic energy pattern maintains sufficient of the original for us to experience the message it contains. This message can carry information which stimulates us as individuals, mentally, emotionally, and physically. It can stimulate us to think, to be happy or sad, or to laugh or cry. Similarly, the message carried in homeopathic remedies from the original source, can stimulate us on all of these levels.

However, the remedy must bring appropriate information to the individual if it is to have any effect. This is why it is necessary to select the appropriate remedy for the individual. To use our previous example, the voice of someone you recognize/love may have a profound effect on you, while leaving others unmoved. The effect is not transferable or reproducible in others, because individuals are different.

The homeopathic remedy acts as information. This stimulates the body to respond with its own powers of self-healing; mental, emotional and physical. Unlike orthodox medicines, the remedies have little or no chemical content depending on their level of dilution. This means that unlike other medicines, they cannot give rise to toxic side-effects that accumulate in the body. In fact, they are so safe that they are routinely used in pregnancy, and also for babies and young children, with no fear of side-effects. Neither is there any risk of addiction or dependency.

THE ROLE OF THE MIND

Y our mind, like your body, is a combination of inherited and acquired characteristics. While we are aware of the way in which physical illness can affect our mental state, for example, pain may lead us to be irritable or depressed, we often overlook the fact that this works both ways. In fact, our mental and emotional state is very clearly linked to disease (dis-ease). Our habitual mental and emotional states and attitudes, can over a period of time result in predictable, physical diseases. Homeopathic and other holistic therapists have worked with this knowledge for centuries. Now psycho-neuro-immunology is beginning to look at how this takes place.

The body appears to compensate for our unbalanced mental or emotional state by creating the opposite condition. Individuals who demand too much performance from themselves without knowing when to say no, may develop ME. Some-one who maintains extreme control for most of his or her life may develop Parkinson's disease where all control is lost. Someone unable to face the present or future may retreat into Alzheimer's disease.

Simplistic? Yes, but it happens, even though we are only just starting to recognize it, let alone understand the process whereby long-held attitudes manifest as physical dis-ease.

One of the things that holds us back is our reluctance to accept responsibility for our mental and physical health. It is currently more acceptable to be a victim, but that takes away our power. And our minds do have the power to affect our bodies. We do it all the time with only a thought. Fold your arms, there you did it! Think an embarrassing thought and blush. You did it again! Think of something frightening and see your pulse rate soar. We can control our bodies, and when we accept that we all play a part, albeit an unwitting one in the creation of our dis-ease, we can begin to un-create the conditions that led us to our current state, whatever that is.

The downside is that however hard it is to change physical habits and addictions, like the choice not to smoke any more, it is much, much harder to change our habitual negative thought patterns and beliefs, no matter how much harm they do to us over the years. Half the time we are not even aware of them, or willing to discuss them, let alone change them. We would rather die, and sometimes literally do. But then even with the best will in the world it is still very hard.

If you are anxious you may know that it is not doing you any good, but it does not make it any easier to stop. If you push yourself too hard you may know it is killing you but you have probably got 101 reasons why you have to do it. If you are lucky enough to have some warning symptoms, do not ignore them, do not suppress them, decide to change for the better.

Illness is like a fuse. If illness tells you to stop, take stock, do not just replace the fuse and wait for the problem to recur, or try to weave round it and create a much more dangerous situation. Try to figure out what the real problem is and work at changing it. This is when homeopathic treatment can help so much. It can help you to rebalance mentally and emotionally, and support you through the whole process, as well as helping you physically.

This is why homeopathic, and other holistic therapists, treat the patient on all levels whenever possible. Only in this way, is a true and lasting cure possible, rather than merely stopping the dis-ease producing warning symptoms, by using surgery or ongoing drugging. For if we just suppress physical symptoms without addressing their cause then the problem will return.

If, for example, you stop some of the physical symptoms that can result from ongoing stress, without either removing the stress or enabling the individual to cope with it in a less damaging way, you merely create more serious symptoms in the future. Homeopathic treatment seeks to restore the health of the whole individual (mental/emotional and physical), and by removing inherited and acquired miasms (tendencies towards illness), to ensure that they stay healthy.

HOW THE REMEDIES ARE MADE

Alcohol is used to extract the active ingredients from the source of each remedy. The resulting ticture is then carefully diluted and succussed (shaken) to potentise it. This is repeated as many times as necessary to make the desired potency. For example, one drop of tincture to nine drops of water makes a 1× potency. If one drop of this is taken, added to nine more drops of water and shaken, then a 2× potency has been created. Similarly, 1 C is created by adding one drop of tincture to 99 drops of water, taking one drop of this solution and adding it to a further 99 drops of water to create the 2C potency, and so on up the scale. Each succession adds more energy (potency) to the remedy even though it is increasingly diluted.

The resulting liquids are called medicating potencies and are then dropped onto small white lactose or sucrose tablets or pillules for ease of taking. Soft tablets can be used for babies and toddlers, or one drop of medicating liquid itself can be placed on to the tongue or rubbed onto the skin (e.g. navel). Powders may also be used or a hard tablet can be crushed between 2 teaspoons. Remedies made from various forms of radiation are produced by leaving lactose powder exposed to the source of the radiation for several hours before potentizing by dilution and succussion in the normal way.

3
• • • • •

Using Symptoms to Find the Right Remedy

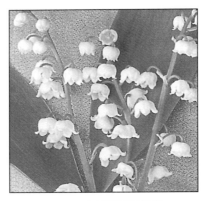

LILLEY OF THE VALLEY
Source of the homeopathic remedy
Convallaria majalis

We have thousands of homeopathic remedies to choose from; and many different strengths (the potency) for each remedy. Unlike conventional medicine, we cannot just look up the name of a disease and select from a few drugs to treat that disease. We are treating the patient! So we have to ask, what started your health problem (often this is only apparent from probing questions, as there may be a delay of two years or more between the cause and the effect)? How does this asthma affect you? When or what makes it better, what makes it worse? Thus, the more information you are able to give your homeopath, the quicker and more effectively she/he will be able to help you.

What does it feel like to you? Perhaps you assume that your headache is like my headache. That is very unlikely when you consider that in one homeopathic reference book alone there are 1,824 different categories of headache listed, with a different group of remedies listed for each type of headache. It is the job of the homeopath to choose the relevant entries for your type of headache and then select the most appropriate remedy from those listed, by considering other factors such as when and how your headaches began, and what sort of person you are (your constitutional make-up).

We are often out of touch with our feelings – both emotional and physical. I ask patients how does this event make you *feel*. Instead, they will start to tell me what they *think*. The two things are very different. We can often make an unpleasant experience second-hand and safe by thinking it over rather than exploring how it actually made us feel. When patients express thoughts, rationalizations, judgements and reflections it can be interesting and tell us something about their intellect and influences.

However, when we say how something made/makes us feel we are in touch with a very real and deep part of ourselves. If the experience was traumatic or painful, the eyes may fill with tears. It very quickly becomes obvious to the practitioner and the patient (who is sometimes unaware) just how much they were affected by an event, and how it may have impacted on their health even many years later.

Similarly, in the same book mentioned previously, there are 26,746 references to physical pain, each with their own group of useful remedies. Yet when you ask some patients to describe their pain, to aid in the selection of a remedy, they will find it difficult. 'Oh I try not to dwell upon that.' All very heroic, but the pain and more particularly its nature, origin, extent, frequency, duration and what alleviates and aggravates it, is there to tell us what is wrong; and more importantly for the homeopath, how to put it right.

So we need to be in touch with our feelings, both emotional and physical. How did that make us feel? Were we resentful, angry, hurt, sad, desolate, anxious or fearful? What does the pain feel like? Is it shooting, throbbing, bruised, stinging, stabbing, aching, dull, sharp, tearing, pressing, piercing, hammering, burning, sore, drawing?, etc. etc. We need to be in touch with ourselves physically and emotionally in order to halt and reverse serious ongoing health problems. This is not always easy as our problems often begin from a lack of awareness or suppression of our emotional and/or physical needs.

Some remedies work well on particular organs, or particular parts of the body. It is important to consider exactly where the sensation is felt. Does the sensation stay in one place? If it is in our head, then where exactly is it located? Is the feeling over our eyes, or behind them. Is it just on the left side, or does it start on the left and move to the right? Is the sensation focused in a small spot, or does it extend to another part of the body? The answers to all these questions and more, will help us to find the best remedy.

We may have the same complaint as our neighbour, but what makes *our* problem worse? Is it aggravated by sunlight, or perhaps it is worse when it is windy? Our neighbour on the other hand, may be much better for sunshine, but worse for any movement. Taking these symptoms into account, the two of us will most likely need different remedies. It is this individualization and attention to detail that is at the heart of true homeopathic prescription.

4
•••••

Homeopathy and Orthodox Medicine

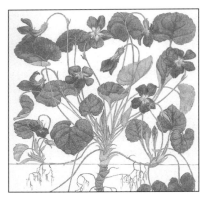

VIOLET
Source of the homeopathic remedy
Viola odorata

T he advantages are obvious. Cheap, effective
medicine with no side-effects. This is why
homeopathy has been so widely used throughout
the world during the past two hundred years or
more. It is also why homeopathy is the only so-
called complementary medicine to be available

under Britain's National Health Service since it began in 1948.

Homeopathic remedies are cheap to produce and they sell cheaply. So why bother with crude drugs at all?

A common argument against using homeopathy more widely is lack of reproducible trials. However, reproducible trials as defined by orthodox scientific and medical practice are inappropriate to apply to homeopathy. You cannot give a hundred people the same homeopathic remedy for asthma and expect excellent results, because the whole essence of homeopathy is an individualized prescription. The remedy or series of remedies, must be very carefully chosen on the basis of a painstaking matching process. The remedies must match the particular symptoms of the patient rather than the disease. In fact, any symptoms common to all patients with asthma, are the least important ones to consider when it comes to finding the most effective homeopathic treatment for a particular asthma sufferer.

In spite of this, a randomized controlled trial of homeopathy versus placebo in perennial allergic rhinitis, which was reported in the *BMJ* (*British Medical Journal*) on 19–26 August 2000 showed that '. . . those in the homeopathic group had significantly greater improvements in *objective* measurement of nasal airflow than did the placebo group'.

One of the reasons why a homeopath needs to spend more time with a patient than an allopathic doctor, is that we take into account all your symptoms. By contrast, an allopathic doctor generally confines himself to what you say is your main complaint. Through diagnosis, a label can be put on what is wrong with you, and you can be given the current drug treatment for that condition, or referred to a specialist, who may then focus even more on one particular aspect of your health.

In the often limited time which an allopathic doctor has to spend with her/his patients, it is natural to concentrate on the part of the body which is causing most problems and ignore the rest. Homeopathic treatment differs in that it is usually based on an holistic approach. This means that we gather as much information as possible about the patient. We see each individual as a unique and whole being. Treatment is based on the sum of information about a patient. The unique combination of symptoms for each patient determines our unique treatment and choice of remedies for that patient.

For example, patients A and B both want treatment to stop recurring migraine headaches. On further questioning, patient A says that that he is suffering from mouth ulcers, hot sweaty hands, a cracked lower lip and indigestion. Although we have hundreds of homeopathic remedies from which we can choose to cure migraine, on the basis of these additional symptoms we know that the remedy Natrum Mur is likely to be especially useful.

On the other hand, patient B tells us that in addition to his migraine headaches, he suffers from mental fatigue, problems with memory, and an enlarged prostate gland. Using these symptoms, we would consider the remedy Lycopodium.

Of course, these additional symptoms are still only part of the total picture. In reality, a final choice will be based on consideration of the specific sensations of each patient's migraine, the particular location of any head pain, and what makes it better or worse etc.

One of the joys of homeopathy, is that because the remedy is chosen to improve the whole patient, these additional symptoms, which an allopathic doctor may not even be aware of, are likely to disappear along with the migraine. Not only that, the patient often reports that an additional symptom which they forgot to mention to you, has has disappeared after all these years.

☐

Once drugs were the alternative. Now, thanks to very successful marketing, they are mainstream, although our love affair with them has worn off. We know that antibiotics are useless for viruses and that steroids have serious side-effects. Allopathy (mainstream orthodox medicine) encourages us to think of anything else as complementary, thus safeguarding its own existence. Well, homeopathy can be complementary in that it can improve the patient's overall health when allopathic treatment is also being given. However, for many patients it is a preferable alternative (See case histories in Chapter 6 for some examples).

5 .....

Understanding Illness and Healing

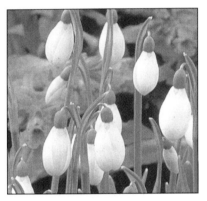

SNOWDROPS
Source of the homeopathic remedy
Galanthus nivalis

Homeopathy is not just about stopping symptoms. The quickest way to stop your symptoms is to kill you! In fact, symptoms are produced by the body to help you! But how can feeling awful help me, you may say? Pain alerts you to the fact that something is wrong, and we need to take action to make the situation (not primarily the pain) better. Take care of the problem and the pain will take care of itself. Similarly, a rise in temperature, is part of the healing process, speeding the chemical reactions which are working away *feverishly* to get you better. It also has the added bonus that it makes you feel lousy so you are more likely to rest, which will further aid recovery. That is unless you sabotage your own built-in repair system by taking something to get rid of your symptoms so you can carry on regardless!

Reduce the swelling – why? Swelling protects the site of injury while your body sends healing fluids to the damaged tissues. Vomiting, and maybe diarrhoea, is the body's intelligent response to being poisoned. A speedy and helpful response to an unhealthy situation. Not merely an outcome of the illness and certainly not something to be suppressed.

The view that the body invariably responds in the best, most helpful way possible, in order to attempt to restore a balanced state of health to the individual, is one of the main differences in approach to illness between homeopathy and conventional medicine. Homeopathic remedies support the inherent, natural, healing responses of the individual; conventional drugs work in opposition to this process to suppress symptoms.

A homeopath uses your symptoms to select treatment that will deal with the *underlying cause of those symptoms*. That is why you usually do not need to take homeopathic remedies long-term, unlike most conventional treatment where symptoms can recur as soon as you stop the drugs, simply because nothing has been changed; symptoms were merely suppressed for as long as you continued with the drugs.

Homeopathy asserts that true healing of the whole individual (not just odd symptoms):

- Starts from the top of the body and works downward.
- Starts from within the body working outwards towards the surface, and from major to minor organs.

And that

- Your most recent symptoms will disappear first followed by ones you have had longer (i.e. in the reverse order to their onset).

Homeopathic treatment is, therefore, based on the whole individual, including inherited factors and acquired mental, emotional and physical characteristics. The exception to this is therapeutic or first aid homeopathic treatment for acute rather than chronic illness. This type of treatment is useful for everyday complaints such as cuts, burns, bruises, broken bones, crushing injuries etc. It is particularly suitable for self-treatment (see Chapter 7 for more details).

☐

Why is it that we do not all get the same illnesses? I tend to suffer from stomach problems. You have chest problems, perhaps a tendency for colds to develop into bronchitis, or perhaps you suffer from asthma. The meningitis bug is all around and inside us but only the 'unlucky' ones succumb. Why? The answer is that illness is an outcome of the relationship between our personal constitution or make-up and our environment.

Homeopathy can help you even if you are relatively healthy. Through constitutional treatment we aim to make you less susceptible to those illnesses to which you tend to fall prey. However, the stresses, strains, pollution etc. of living in the twenty-first century will gradually aggravate your built-in weaknesses, to a greater or lesser extent depending on your particular constitution. Further constitutional homeopathic treatment periodically, together with a healthy life-style will help to reduce your susceptibility to illness.

OUR ACHILLES HEELS (MIASMS)

You inherited your constitution, together with certain weaknesses that were created in previous generations, and passed down to you. These are known as *miasms*, which we can call our Achilles heels. Frequently, they are the leftover effects of our ancestors, exposure to such maladies as tuberculosis, gonorrhoea and syphilis. We, in turn, add to our inherited susceptibilities (miasms), new, acquired susceptibilities/weaknesses (acquired miasms), or through suppression of our symptoms rather than cure, we turn old illnesses into new ones. And so it goes on, each generation passing on its bundle of genetic material and viruses (often dormant) to the next.

Homeopathic treatment at its deepest level, aims to resolve this. In effect, it tries to 'wipe the slate clean' for current and future generations. Of course, even if it were possible to completely remove inherited miasms, we all periodically acquire new ones in our lifetime. These are the effects on us as individuals of such things as new partners who potentially pass on some of their miasmatic burden to us. Also, the effects of pollution from toxins and radiation in our environment. This is why periodic ongoing homeopathic treatment is of such value in maintaining health.

Sadly, even today, many people still suffer for months or years before seeking out homeopathy as a last resort, rather than using it as a tool for maintaining a good level of health throughout their life. Without treatment, the end result is a worsening of incremental disease patterns over the generations, depending on the prevalent miasms. So, for example, one family may see skin problems deteriorate through suppressive treatment into lung problems such as asthma; another may see physical symptoms appear to clear up, when in fact the expression of the miasm has moved to a deeper and more serious level, expressing itself in clinical depression or even self-destructive behaviour.

This situation dramatically worsened during the latter part of the twentieth century because it appears that while childhood illnesses in otherwise healthy individuals actually help the child to throw off these miasms, the current trend of vaccination not only prevents this natural process from occurring, it makes dormant or mild miasmatic illness dramatically worse! The result is epidemics of asthma, allergies, glue ear etc., as well as the evolution of new diseases such as Aids and later in life, dramatically increased rates of cancer, in spite of all the funding for research and technology.

6

• • • • •

Eight Case Studies

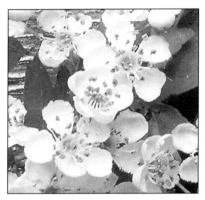

HAWTHORN BLOSSOM
Source of the homeopathic remedy
Crataegus oxyacamtha et monogyna

CASE 1: MENOPAUSAL COMPLAINTS

Like a great many other women, Jean, a retired nurse, came to see me because she was concerned about symptoms she was experiencing due to the menopause. Jean's main problem was uncontrollable and distressing sweats which had started after a hysterectomy. Originally, these had been controlled by HRT (hormone replacement therapy). However, Jean had been taken off HRT the previous year in order to have a mastectomy. Since then she had suffered from between twelve and twenty sweats each day, and on average six at night. The sweats lasted about two minutes, and completely drained her. I spent an hour during the first consultation, taking details of Jean's family medical history, and drawing up a time line of Jean's own medical history. This would come in useful for treating Jean's overall health and susceptibility to illness later on.

To start with, I wanted to give Jean a remedy that would help her, as quickly as possible, to stop sweating. This type of therapeutic treatment is often very useful in providing quick relief to patients who are desperate. Deeper, more holistic constitutional and miasmatic treatment can then follow. Jean was prescribed two remedies to alternate. These were homeopathic preparations of the mineral Sulphur and the plant Nux vomica, both in very low potency.

At our next consultation Jean told me she was not sweating at all on most days, and the worst she had suffered were a couple of mild sweats. In her own words: 'it's absolutely amazing'.

I went on to treat Jean constitutionally – in particular, for a grief that she had never really dealt with – as well as multiple sclerosis from which she had suffered for nearly thirty years. After receiving constitutional treatment Jean's energy improved dramatically. She found that she became less constipated, needed less rest during the day, became less fatigued, and was able to launch herself into spring-cleaning (even though it was late July)!

CASE 2: RHEUMATOID ARTHRITIS

B arry was on sick leave when he came to see me. He had suffered badly with rheumatoid arthritis for the past six years. Anti-inflammatory drugs had helped to control the symptoms for three years, but Barry had stopped them a month previously, due to side-effects, particularly digestive problems.

When he came for treatment he was experiencing a great deal of pain in his shoulders, hands, arms and feet, also stiffness in his knees. He had difficulty going to sleep because of the pain, and walking was difficult. Barry was given Rhus tox, a plant remedy of great help in muscle aches and pains. When I saw him two weeks later his hands had improved, and he told me life was now worth living.

After another two weeks Barry found walking was easier, especially going downstairs. However, he was having trouble sleeping because of severe pain in his right shoulder.

Another two weeks and Barry's hands were still improving, his shoulder was fine, and although he was still feeling a slight discomfort while walking, he had managed to walk over six miles the previous Sunday! With further homeopathic treatment and a change of diet, Barry was able to resume work. He continued to improve, although he still experienced some swelling and pain in his right hand and wrist.

Very often the first symptoms which appear in a patient, are the last to disappear; as healing progresses in the reverse order to that in which the symptoms first appeared.

CASE 3: COPING WITH DEPRESSION & ANXIETY

W hen Graham came to see me, there did not really seem to be much, if anything, wrong with him. However, his family had noticed a difference, and they suggested that he come for treatment. Graham himself told me that he was feeling negative, which was very unlike his normal self. In fact, it soon became clear that he had got stuck, and given time it was likely that his negativity would have turned into depression.

Graham told me that on the surface, everything in his life seemed fine, and yet he felt as if he was walking under a cloud. 'Everything winds me up,' he told me. 'I have always bottled things up, and now I'm worse, I seem to have completely lost my confidence.'

Graham was worried about money and work. He was frustrated with his job, which he said he had only taken as a fill-in, and he admitted to a pattern of wayward decisions, spending six months here, and six months there, before moving on. He was feeling very discontent, and it was obvious that he had experienced this in the past, which had led to him moving on. He was trying to understand why he had this pattern of behaviour, and admitted to crazy ambitious ideas.

Not that there is anything wrong with having ambition, or the odd crazy idea. However, in Graham's case, there was a pattern of not following through with his ideas, but quickly becoming discontent and moving on rather than staying the course. Graham was dissatisfied with the present, but he was not fully living in it. Instead, he was looking back over the past, and regretting the friends he had left behind. At other times he was looking into the future, asking himself what if, and raising all sorts of anxieties/doubts and insecurity which he brought into the present.

Like all of us, Graham had created his present, and it was not a healthy one. He told me: 'I feel boring.' He was very aware that things were not right, but the harder he tried to put things right, the worse things became. He felt he was trying too hard, and being too intense. He summed it up by saying: 'I have gradually lost my smile over the last six months to a year.'

What Graham needed, above all, was spontaneity. But you cannot gain spontaneity by being intense and trying too hard. He was not enjoying life, because he was living in past regrets, and future anxieties. Fortunately, the prognosis was good, because Graham was aware of what was happening to him and determined to get back on track. All that was needed to start the process was a single dose of the appropriate miasmatic remedy in high potency.

Ten days later, Graham came to see me, feeling fine. He told me that it was quite bizarre the way that his life had turned around in the last ten days. People had suddenly become more interested in him and what he had to say, and he was making new friends. He told me: 'I feel a lot better in myself'. This is one of the most important signs that a remedy is working to re-balance the individual and return them to a healthier, more harmonious state. In fact, Graham was feeling so positive that he decided he was going to give up smoking, and asked me for some remedies which he knew would help him resist addiction, and reduce the effects of nicotine withdrawal.

Another fourteen days, and Graham told me that things were now really going his way again, and he was still making new friends. Graham was given his constitutional remedy in a single high potency dose. This prescription was based on the type of person he was when he was in a healthy state, and designed to return him to that healthy state, mentally, emotionally and physically. The remedy was chosen from the details that Graham had given me originally about his food and drink likes, dislikes and aggravations, weather likes, dislikes and aggravations, as well as his natural emotional behaviour and physical complaints and weaknesses.

During our final consultation, life was still sweet for Graham. His energy was much better, and he had even started up a football team. He was back on course!

CASE 4: CANCER

H omeopaths treat people not diseases. Often the first help needed by people who have just been told that they have cancer, is with the shock and anxiety caused by the diagnosis. With some slow-to-develop forms of cancer, the only treatment option offered by orthodox medicine is monitoring every six months or so, in order to check that the cancer process has not speeded up or the disease spread to other parts of the body. This can often leave the patient feeling very helpless, anxious, and let down. Not the sort of state to help the body regain health. Homeopathic treatment at this stage can do a great deal to help patients to cope with anxiety, fear and depression.

Very often I will be asked by the patient, should I accept the offer of radiotherapy, chemotherapy, surgery etc., or should I concentrate all my efforts on using natural, alternative approaches? It is natural for patients to seek advice, but it is important that ultimately they take responsibility for their choice of treatment. The best a homeopath can do, is to discuss the various options, and the different ways that homeopathy can support the patient whatever they choose.

It is noted by some observers that individuals prone to cancer are often keen to please those around them. In much the same way, the study has recently shown that some particularly cynical individuals seem to be prone to heart problems. I have seen cancer patients agonizing over their choice of treatment, carrying on a pattern of putting themselves last, even though it is their lives that are in the balance.

After exploring and evaluating the pros and cons of surgery or chemotherapy, they may often conclude that they do not want those forms of drastic intervention. However, their loved ones often see the orthodox way as their best chance. In spite of not being comfortable with the idea of orthodox treatment, the patient will again put their own feelings second, and choose to do what will please the family, even to the point where they believe that their chances of surviving will be reduced by their decision.

Even in their time of need their choice is often made on the basis of a sacrifice for the needs of others which they put first. However, the fact that this often becomes apparent to them during the course of homeopathic treatment, can help them to recognize for the first time, a tendency to suppress their own needs, which can then start a process leading to them taking better care of themselves in future. Whatever path is chosen, homeopathic treatment can be invaluable. The following case study shows how homeopathy can be used in conjunction with conventional treatment – in this case, chemotherapy.

☐

A lice is an elderly lady who came to see me having just been diagnosed with cancer of the ovary and intestine. She had gone into hospital three weeks previously for an operation to remove the tumour. However, the surgeon had found that the tumour had spread too far for surgery to be effective. So nothing was removed; instead, Alice was instead offered chemotherapy and a possible further operation at some point in the future. She had only returned home from hospital one week prior to me visiting her at home. Still weak from the operation, Alice's weight had dropped to six stones (84 pounds), and she was suffering from a prolapse, severe indigestion and also incontinence following the removal of a catheter. Just before Christmas, I spent about an hour and a half with Alice, taking full details of her medical history as well as details of her family's medical history.

The first remedy I gave Alice was Staphisagria to deal with the immediate problem of her incontinence, while I worked out the most appropriate treatment to support her overall health. Naturally, Alice was very anxious about her condition and future treatment. This anxiety was interfering with her sleep, and because lack of sleep would put additional stress on her system, this needed to be dealt with.

Commonly, one of the first prescriptions for patients who have just been diagnosed as suffering from a serious illness, is given to help them to deal with the shock, grief, trauma and anxiety which they are likely to experience. This is not in place of listening to the patient, and helping them explore these issues, but rather the remedies needed to support the process of change through which the patient moves towards healing. That it is not to say that the same remedies are used in each case, but as always in homeopathy, we seek out the most appropriate remedy for the individual, based on the totality of the symptoms, their medical history, and what they are like in their healthy state.

Alice was given Arsenicum album, a homeopathic preparation of arsenic trioxide. In potency (when diluted and sucussed), the remedy is completely non-toxic, but still very powerful. The potency used in this case was 30c.

Medium and low potencies are often used when a patient is in a frail, weak state with little energy, as higher potencies may demand too much from the patient, resulting in extreme weariness.

Alice's main reason for choosing homeopathy, stemmed from her concern about the side-effects of chemotherapy. Although she had decided to receive chemotherapy, she felt that homeopathy would help her through the process. Her first treatment was scheduled for one week into the New Year. About a week before this, she started taking a combination of homeopathic remedies chosen to help her organs deal more effectively with the toxins used in chemotherapy, with the aim of reducing side-effects.

☐

O ver the next year, Alice had twelve chemotherapy treatments in total. She continued to take a combination of organ support remedies, and in addition further remedies were prescribed for problems that came up during the course of her orthodox treatment. Examples of specific problems which arose, many of which were very distressing, were restless legs, frequent need to urinate, dyspepsia, severe constipation, flatulence, distension, nausea, and vomiting, hair loss, sleeplessness, pain, frequent need to pass a stool, low haemoglobin (requiring blood transfusion), numbness and pins and needles, thrush (following antibiotic treatment), low white blood cell count and resulting fever. Throughout her treatment Alice took homeopathic remedies daily. These were prescribed with the constant aim of reducing the physical problems she was experiencing, and supporting her mentally and emotionally.

Six months into this ordeal, and after six chemotherapy treatments, Alice had to decide whether she could face starting a second course of chemotherapy using new and more toxic drugs, which her body had not originally been strong enough to cope with. She decided to continue with both orthodox treatment and homeopathic treatment.

The good news is, that nearly a year later, following all of this treatment, a very courageous lady has been told that her tumour has shrunk to a quarter of its original size! Treatment will continue, and even after orthodox treatment stops, there will still be much left for homeopathy to contribute in its attempt to aid the patient to achieve the healthiest state possible for her.

CASE 5: CHILDREN'S COMPLAINTS – GLUE EAR/ECZEMA

M any children are brought to me after being given four or more courses of antibiotics in less than two months. Not only is the original problem recurring at the end of every course, the child is now far more susceptible to illness as a result of the antibiotics weakening the body's own defence system. Homeopathy can quickly deal with conditions such as sore throats and earaches – as you will find in Chapter 7 on the self-treatment. However, it can take longer to restore the individual through constitutional and miasmatic treatment, to the point where they are no longer susceptible to repeated attacks.

☐

A ndrew was four years old when he was brought to see me suffering from glue ear. In spite of four recent courses of antibiotics, he was frequently suffering from painful earache and experiencing hearing problems. Andrew had had the ear problems since birth, but because of a slight heart murmur his parents were keen to avoid him having grommets fitted under general anaesthetic. Andrew was also asthmatic, which was controlled with orthodox drugs.

After just two doses of Pulsatilla 30c, Andrew's earache cleared up, 'quicker than using any other medicine'. I also gave him a dose of Thuja to deal with any aggravation to his miasmatic weakness' that may have resulted from vaccinations in the past. He was then given single doses of two miasmatic remedies to deal with his inherited susceptibility to these types of malady, as well as Lobelia 6X three times a day to help with his breathing, and Aconite to deal with an occasional croupy cough.

After just six weeks, Andrew no longer needed to use either of his inhalers, and his breathing was fine. Much to his delight, and that of his parents, he could now even go swimming again, without wheezing. Not only had his earache been dealt with, but Andrew was off steroids and breathing freely, and his energy had improved dramatically, all in the space of six weeks!

□

C live was brought to see me suffering from eczema. He was four months old and had had the condition since the age of six weeks. As is common in these cases, there was a family history of hay fever, asthma and eczema. Also not unusual was the fact that Clive had had a worsening of his condition after receiving vaccinations.

After his first vaccination at the age of eight weeks, Clive's parents did not notice any aggravation. However, after vaccination at twelve weeks they did notice deterioration. By the time of his third vaccination at sixteen weeks, there was a very clear reaction in the form of an increase in temperature, a rash and general worsening of the skin condition; and as parents often observe, he was far less happy and good-tempered.

Before his third vaccination, Clive's doctor had prescribed hydrocortisone cream. At best this could suppress the skin symptoms, while in my opinion, driving the problem deeper. However, as is often the case, little relief, if any, was gained. The eczema became weepy and appeared to be infected. Then when cream was applied topically, it appeared to spread the eczema. Stopping dairy products, did seem to give some improvement, but Clive's condition worsened considerably after his third vaccination and he was prescribed a course of antibiotics. Further complications were a suspected kidney/bladder problem (picked up by ultrasound scan), for which Clive had already been given antibiotics. He was also just beginning teething.

The number one remedy to help with teething problems is Chamomilla 30c, especially where the child is irritable and wants to be picked up but cannot be pacified. (See Chapter 8 for more information.)

I began Clive's treatment with a miasmatic prescription, aimed at dealing with the susceptibilities and over-sensitivity, which he had inherited from his parents. As well as eczema on his father's side, Clive's mother had been diagnosed with scabies during pregnancy and again ten days after he was born. This was followed over the next few months by homeopathic remedies such as sulphur, and Graphites, as well as homeopathic constitutional treatment. Other remedies used were Tissue Salts (very low potency homeopathic remedies produced from substances which also occur naturally in the body), drainage remedies (to help with the elimination of toxins) and organ support remedies for the bladder, kidneys and skin.

Clive's recovery was slow and patchy. As usual in skin cases, it was necessary to proceed carefully to avoid any aggravation of a problem that was already very distressing to a four-month-old baby and his mother. In addition, Clive was still receiving some orthodox treatment, which on the occasions that it was successful in suppressing the eczema, succeeded in shifting the problem to his lungs, resulting in coughs and wheezing.

Clive's mum persevered with his treatment, trying as much as she could to avoid the use of antibiotics and wet wrapping with steroid cream. Instead, she used moisturizing cream and excluded dairy products and wheat from her diet (these were passing to Clive through her breast milk and aggravating his condition).

A variety of soothing natural creams can be used such as Calendula, Aloe Vera or Stellaria, but it is important to try these out on a small area first, as different individuals respond differently to the creams. These topical applications will not heal the body, but they can make a life more bearable while the homeopathic remedies work from the inside. Many people find that Tea Tree oil can be used to prevent the eczema from becoming infected.

After four or five months, progress was considerable. However, it is very difficult for parents to resist the calls for stronger medication and the continued use of antibiotics and steroids to suppress the symptoms. None of us, particularly the parents, wants to see a child suffer. There is no doubt that it is much easier to resort to steroids, and put up with the potentially much more serious condition of asthma, than to see your child suffer and at the same time be criticized by family and friends for not stopping their symptoms as soon as possible. Unfortunately, their well-meant, but poorly informed comments, can drive parents back to a quick-fix, at the expense of their child's future health.

Parents who can no longer resist the 'quick-fix' pressure may get fewer sleepless nights, and get grandparents off their backs; and besides, who will connect the decision to suppress skin symptoms with the respiratory symptoms which follow? Using powerful drugs to suppress skin symptoms often results in the appearance of respiratory problems such as hay fever, wheezing or asthma; or the worsening of pre-existing respiratory problems. However, parents who persevere towards a homeopathic cure are eventually rewarded with a healthier child.

CASE 6: PROSTATE PROBLEMS

R obert's problem was one that many men feel embarrassed to seek help about. Namely, problems with the prostate gland. He had been diagnosed as having prostadynia. His symptoms began four years ago with an occasional ache in the region of his prostate gland. Gradually, this worsened, until it became at best a continual dull ache, and at worst flaring up into a severe pain that could last for weeks. The constant pain had led to problems with depression. No treatment had ever helped to relieve the pain.

In this case there was no inflammation of the prostate gland, just pain. Treatment commenced with a series of remedies known for their usefulness in prostate conditions, given in low potency. Next time Robert came for treatment, about a month later, he reported that there had been no improvement. The prescription was changed to Hypericum, a very useful remedy for damage to nerves and the resulting pain. After a fortnight taking the remedy in low potency three times a day, the pain got slightly worse. Robert stopped taking the remedy for a day and a half before noticing an improvement. The pain no longer felt so intense, and he felt better in himself. He was advised to continue taking the remedy until I saw him again.

The next time Robert attended the clinic, the pain was completely disappearing for days at a time. He saw this as a great improvement as it had never happened before. To finish the treatment the potency of the Hypericum was increased, and Robert was given a bottle of the remedy in case the pain returned in future.

I should point out that Hypericum was chosen because of Robert's past medical history, taking into account a car accident in his teens and a subsequent back problem. The fact that the remedy helped Robert, does not mean that it would be the appropriate remedy for everyone diagnosed with the same condition.

HYPERICUM – ST JOHN'S WORT

The common name for Hypericum is St Johns' Wort. As well as being very useful where there is damage to nerves, perhaps by crushing, or penetration of a sharp instrument, it is also widely used in a low potency (or as a herbal preparation) to relieve depression.

There have been recent claims that using Hypericum in herbal form can alter the effectiveness of other medications such as the pill. Further research may reveal whether this is more of a problem with Hypericum than any other combination of medicines, or just another scare story protecting the market for tranquilizers and anti – depressant drugs.

At present, there is absolutely no indication that the use of Hypericum homeopathically is likely to cause any problems. However, if you are concerned then consult a qualified homeopath.

CASE 7: PREGNANCY AND CHILDBIRTH FOR THE OLDER WOMAN

Alison had her last baby almost twenty years ago. Finding that she was pregnant again after all those years was a roller-coaster of emotions, heightened by the hormonal changes occurring as her body remembered what to do to accommodate the precious new life growing inside her.

Her previous baby had been born by caesarean section after a failed induction. This time she was determined to take this last chance to have a natural birth. Alison had cranial osteopathy during the pregnancy in order to rectify a hip misalignment. Knowing that homeopathic remedies are totally safe to use during pregnancy, she followed my standard program of treatment.

This program is designed to increase the elasticity of the skin and tissue in order to avoid stretch marks, to counter anaemia (without the use of iron supplements which may encourage bleeding), to reduce the risk of haemorrhaging, to help deal with nervous exhaustion, to tone the uterus and to reduce muscle cramps.

In this case it was felt to be particularly important to tone the uterus, because of possible weakness in the area of previous caesarean surgery.

In addition, Alison was given remedies to help her with the emotional conflict, trauma and grief which occurred as it became clear that there was a slight possibility that her baby had Down's syndrome, and she sought to decide whether to find out from an amniocentesis test (which could damage the developing foetus) or to accept her baby whatever the final outcome.

Alison eventually decided that while she felt she could still love and care for her baby even if he/she had special needs, she would not be able to live with the grief that would ensue if her unborn baby was damaged during an amniocentesis.

Alison arrived at the hospital at about 1.00 am on a Sunday morning. She had her first examination by the midwife at 2.30 am and was found to be 4 cm dilated. Estimated time of arrival for 'Louise' was 10.30 am. At 2.30 am the midwife unsuccessfully tried to insert a drip needle into the back of Alison's hand. This is done routinely in order give a drug to reduce stomach acidity and reduce the risks from general anaesthetic should it be required at any stage. Arnica 200c was given for bruising.

Five minutes later, Alison was shaking and it was clear that she was in shock. She was given Aconite 200c and the shaking stopped immediately. At 3.15 am a doctor came to insert the drip needle. This was done very efficiently and speedily; however, Alison felt assaulted and angry. Staphysagria 30c was given and she became much more chatty and relaxed straight away. At 3.30 am Hypericum 30c was given for nerve pain caused by the puncture wounds to the hand. At 4.10 am Alison was given Mag. phos. 30c dissolved in water to sip to help with the pain.

At 5.10 am the pain of the contractions was starting to be very uncomfortable so Mag phos. 200c was given. This was used up by one contraction, and therefore was repeated at 5.20 am. It was repeated on demand as the pain increased, at 5.55 am and again at 6.25 am. At 7.00 am the cervix was 6 cms dilated and Caulophyllum was given to speed dilation. As Alison became irritable from the pain of the contractions, Chamomilla 200c was given in place of the Mag. phos. At this point she also tried using gas and air for a short time. However, the gas and air meant that she was unable to keep using her breathing techniques to help during the contractions, so she decided to use only remedies to help with the pain. At 7.50 am the cervix was 9 cm, a change of 3 cm in an hour and fifty minutes! Now just another 4 cms to go and the pushing could begin. Or so we thought.

Suddenly, the baby was becoming distressed. The heartbeat monitor showed that the heart rate was going down during contractions – perhaps the cord was around the neck? Within minutes a foetal blood sample was taken from the baby's head to test the Ph. The results showed that the baby was borderline distressed and it was suggested that a caesarean be performed after all. A final check of the cervix showed that it was not fully dilated, and that instead it was thickening more and more.

By now Alison had had enough, her dream of a natural birth lost in the pain and exhaustion of the last few hours. She was given Chamomilla 200c for the pain and Aconite 200c for her fear. In an attempt to get the cervix to dilate fully, I gave Caulophyllum 12x followed by Caulophyllum 200c five minutes later. Knowing how important a natural birth was to Alison, and with only seconds to spare before the decision to perform a caesarean became inevitable, I switched to Gelsemium 200c. Much to everyone's surprise the cervix disappeared as if by magic. The team were quick to respond and within minutes, at 9.11 am, with the help of an episiotomy and forceps, the registrar pulled, Alison pushed and Louise shot out into the world, over an hour ahead of schedule!

I cut the birth cord and gave mother and baby a dose each of Arnica 200c for the shock and trauma. Louise was just fourteen minutes old when she had her first remedy. Alison then had Staphysagria for bleeding and trauma caused by the episiotomy and Bellis 200c for the internal bruising and damage to soft tissue.

☐

T he labour and birth was a brilliant example of what can be achieved when orthodox medicine and homeopathy work together in harmony to the benefit of the patient. Just six hours later, mother, baby and family were able to go home together to share the joy of their new arrival.

A few days later, news came through confirming that Louise did have Down's syndrome. However, the good news is that a medium-sized hole in her heart has closed after homeopathic and bio-resonance treatment. She is now a thriving, vibrant toddler, who has never needed antibiotics or any other form of allopathic treatment.

CASE 8: ALLERGIES & FOOD INTOLERANCE

M ore and more people are suffering from allergies and food intolerance. But many are confused by the terms.

Allergies
Put simply, the body suffers an allergic response when antibodies attach themselves to harmless foods such as nuts, wheat or dairy products, mistaking them for invading bacteria or viruses. This shows up in a blood test as an increase in the level of Immunoglobin E. Sufferers can experience very violent reactions, leading on occasion to anaphylactic shock, a condition in which the blood pressure plummets while the mouth, tongue and lips swell up. It can be so severe, that unless an antidote

is administered in a form of adrenaline the patient may die.

Food intolerance

Food intolerance, on other hand, differs in that there is no increase in the level of Immunoglobin E. However, the body's sensitivity to certain foods, chemicals or metals can trigger very unpleasant symptoms in the patient. These can range from rashes, digestive problems (such as bloating) and palpitations, to acne, eczema and even asthma. Conventional blood tests will be of no use in identifying the triggers in these cases.

Often food intolerances develop after many years of over-exposure to substances that in more reasonable amounts may not cause us problems. The West is a wheat-based culture, so it comes as little surprise that wheat or gluten is one of the most common culprits. However, whether the problem is caused by wheat, dairy products or something else, with appropriate homeopathic treatment we should, in time, be able to return to a moderate intake of the problem substance.

The beauty of homeopathy in the treatment of allergies and intolerance, is that we do not have to be certain of the trigger, as we can treat an individual's specific symptoms.

There are a variety of tests available, which can suggest possible triggers in the individual (often patients already have a good idea of problem substances). Tests offered include bio-feedback, skin-prick tests, and hair analysis.

☐

H omeopathic treatment can provide therapeutic relief for distressing acute symptoms. However, as always, the aim is to provide a deeper cure. The practitioner may treat the patient constitutionally, to improve their overall level of health, or on an even deeper (miasmatic) level to reduce their inherited susceptibility (i.e. over-sensitivity). Treatment can also be given to desensitize the patient to specific triggers by using the substance in homeopathic form (or by using a remedy that in its crude form would cause similar symptoms). This is completely safe, unlike the allopathic version of desensitization, which resulted in several deaths from anaphylactic shock when it was originally introduced (although it is now said to be safe).

It is interesting to note that recent research from Guy's, King's and St Thomas's School of Medicine in London, reported a link between worsening asthma and frequent use of paracetamol. With ever-growing numbers of young children suffering from asthma, parents may be well advised to check over-the-counter syrups (widely used for pain/teething/colic/fevers etc in babies and infants) for paracetamol! Time and time again, homeopaths see children who suffer eczema or asthma for the first time following vaccinations. Perhaps any aggravation caused by the vaccination is made even worse by the medicinal syrup containing paracetamol, which is often given to reduce the fever that sometimes follows.

The link in these cases is simple: any substance or treatment which interferes with the body's natural defences, may result in a malfunctioning or break-down of the immune system, resulting in an increase in the likelihood of inappropriate reactions to normally harmless substances. Taken on its own, the system can cope with a degree of toxicity. But if a cocktail of vaccination (each containing many different chemicals) is injected into the bloodstream, together with other stressors such as pollution and toxicity from drugs, pesticides and herbicides etc, then we should hardly be surprised when our normally effective defence systems fail or over-react.

BEWARE OF EXCLUSION DIETS

Do be wary of exclusion diets. There is a danger that once the body is free from a number of foods that cause low level chronic symptoms, it can prove very difficult to reintroduce them again. Because an over-sensitive individual will often be affected by several different foods, the result can be that individuals end up restricting their diet to an unsustainable one. If exclusion diets are felt to be necessary, it is sensible to enlist the help of an appropriate medical practitioner.

7 ...
. . . . .

Guidelines for Treating Yourself (AND YOUR PETS)

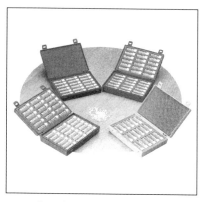

Some homeopathic first-aid kits

WHEN CAN YOU SAFELY TREAT YOURSELF?

Acute illnesses are treatable at home provided that you have access to about thirty or so of the most commonly used homeopathic remedies. By acute, I mean complaints that occur fairly quickly, having clear symptoms, which after a period of time would get better on their own. With very early treatment when you notice the first symptoms, you may be able to stop the complaint developing at all. At the very least, if you select the appropriate remedy, you will reduce the severity of the symptoms and shorten the period of suffering.

Examples of illnesses/conditions which you can treat yourself are colds, flu, coughs, stings, bites, mild cases of childhood diseases (e.g. mumps and chickenpox etc.), bumps and bruises, squashed fingers or toes, sprains, hangovers, travel sickness, earache, toothache etc.

If you cannot find the complaint and/or the symptoms you are looking for in the table of complaints that follows, then contact a professional homeopath for advice/treatment.

Many homeopaths run Homeopathic First-Aid courses. In a few hours' study a week, you can learn how to use remedies such as those listed later in this chapter. You may get to compile your own homeopathic remedy first-aid kit as part of the course, or you could buy a kit of about 18 to 36 of the most frequently used remedies. Remedy kits are easy to carry in a handbag or the glove compartment of a car. You will always have them and therefore not be helpless in a trauma, accident or crisis situation. One day they may even save your life, or that of someone you love. For details of local courses contact your homeopath. Courses may also be found through adult education directories and via the Internet.

WHAT IF THE ACUTE DISEASE IS SERIOUS
OR LIFE-THREATENING?

A s always, use your common sense: if you are concerned, then make a telephone call to your medical practitioner first. However, while you are waiting for help to arrive, the appropriate remedies can be used to great effect. By the time you see your practitioner, the patient may already be over the worst. Correct use of homeopathic remedies at home, can save lives, but never fail to seek professional medical advice when you would normally do so.

For example, you fear that your child may be showing signs of meningitis. In this example, you must immediately telephone your GP or local hospital, but while waiting for help, the patient would benefit very much from the indicated homeopathic remedy, for example, Belladonna or Apis.

After administering homeopathic remedies for acute complaints, patients may improve rapidly. It may be necessary to stress very strongly the seriousness of the original symptoms if an orthodox medical practitioner is called. For example, someone who has fallen downstairs and damaged her spine, may very usefully be given Arnica to help the bruising, shock and trauma. The patient may improve so much that when further help arrives, the seriousness of their injuries is underestimated. Therefore, always stress what happened before the remedies were given, as some orthodox practitioners not familiar with the benefits of homeopathy, might otherwise misread the situation and possibly give inappropriate advice or treatment.

HOW DO I DECIDE WHICH IS THE INDICATED REMEDY?

T o decide which remedy to use, you need to find the remedy which most closely matches the symptoms of the individual with the acute complaint. To enable you to do that, I have listed many of the acute complaints that you may want to treat, together with the remedies that are likely to be most useful. To find the best remedy for your patient, note her/his particular symptoms, find the complaint in the alphabetical list, and choose the remedy whose description best matches the patient's symptoms. In this way, the choice of remedy is individualized to ensure that the most appropriate remedy is given in each case.

Chapter 8 sets out a short Materia Medica. You can use the entries in this section to check further on the suitability of your chosen remedy; or to find out more about the remedy and other uses for it.

WHAT POTENCY SHOULD I TAKE?

M ost homeopathic remedies sold in chemists (drug stores) and health shops are 6c or 30c. As a rough guide try to use the higher potency for things that come on suddenly and for emergencies and accidents. After one or two doses of the appropriate remedy in 30c, you should experience an improvement. At the beginning of an acute attack, take the remedy every hour (more frequently in emergencies) for three or four doses; by which time if you have selected the right remedy, there is likely to be a significant improvement. Continue with the remedy if the improvement shows signs of stopping, taking one to three doses daily, for a few more days (or until improvement has stopped). Always discontinue the remedy when the patient is better or if new symptoms appear.

TREATMENT OF PETS

J ust like us, animals benefit from homeopathic treatment. The main difference is that, like babies and very young children, they cannot tell us what is wrong. Instead, we have to observe them. Farmers and homeopathic veterinarians have successfully treated mastitis in cows for many years using Phytolacca or Belladonna. Horses also are increasingly benefiting from homeopathic remedies for all manner of injuries and complaints. Organic farmers avoid routine use of antibiotics and other drugs by treating their animals using homeopathic remedies. These leave no chemical residues behind to enter the human food chain.

If an animal has the symptoms listed under the remedy then that remedy can be used to help restore health safely. Dosage is the same for pets as for the rest of your family – the 30c potency being the most commonly used for first-aid/acute treatment. You do not need to reduce the potency or dosage for smaller animals/birds/fish etc. Remedies can be dissolved in drinking water or administered into the mouth in tablet form.

All complaints where the symptoms are obvious can be easily treated just by choosing the remedy that matches the symptoms. Obvious examples are sprains, bruises, cuts and scratches, broken bones, abscesses etc. Just use the Table of Complaints which follows, to help you to select the most appropriate remedy.

BEWARE OF THE FOLLOWING SYMPTOMS

You should seek professional help if anyone you are treating has any of the following symptoms:

- DIFFICULTY BREATHING
- HEAVY OR UNEXPECTED BLEEDING
- CONVULSIONS
- FITS
- UNEXPLAINED DROWSINESS
- FEVER ABOVE 40°C OR 103.5°F (ESPECIALLY WITH A STIFF NECK)
- SWELLING OF THE MOUTH OR THROAT
- SEVERE PAINS IN THE CHEST
- SEVERE BURNS

TABLE OF COMPLAINTS WITH REMEDIES

EMERGENCIES

Complaint	Symptoms/cause	Remedies to consider
Bites and stings	Bee, Wasp, Hornet	Aconite, **Apis**, Arnica, Cantharis, Hypericum, **Ledum**
	Dog, Cat, Rat, Horse	Arnica, Belladonna, Hypericum, Ledum
	Mosquito, Gnat, Horsefly	Apis, Cantharis, Hypericum, Ledum
	Jellyfish	Arnica, Hypericum, Ledum
	Snake, Spider, Scorpion	Arnica, Lachesis, Ledum
Bleeding	Small wounds	Arnica, Phosphorus
	After surgery	Phosphorus
Bones	Before setting	Arnica
	Broken (use only after bone is properly set)	Symphytum
	Bruised	Arnica, Ruta, Symphytum
Bruises	General	Arnica, Bellis
	Soft tissue (e.g. breast)	Bellis
	Parts rich in nerves	Hypericum
	Eyeball	Symphytum
Burns and scalds	Rawness and/or blistering	Cantharis
	Shock	Arnica
Crushing injuries	e.g. fingers and toes	Hypericum
Cuts and wounds	Inflamed	Aconite, Apis, Silica
	With pus	Silica
	Lacerated	Calendula
	Punctured (from nails and barbed wire etc.)	**Ledum**, Hypericum
	Splinters	Silica
Frostbite	Bluish skin	Lachesis
	Stinging pain	Apis
Head injuries	Blow to the head	Arnica
Nosebleed	General	Arnica, Ipecac, Lachesis, Phosphorus

Complaint	Symptoms/cause	Remedies to consider
Nosebleed (cont.)	Bright red blood	**Phosphorus**, Ipecac
	Dark blood	Lachesis
	Gushing	Ipecac
Pain	Unbearable	Chamomilla
	Worse from touch	Arnica
	Shooting	**Hypericum**, Belladonna
	Throbbing and hot	Belladonna
	Camping, neuralgic	Mag phos
Shock	General	Arnica
	With fear and restlessness	Aconite
Splinters	Wood, shards of metal or glass, bone etc., **do not use this remedy if you have any implants such as metal pins, pacemaker etc.**	Silica
Sprains and strains	Muscles	Arnica, **Rhus tox**
	Joints	Arnica, Ledum, Rhus tox
	Small joints	Ruta
	Tendons and ligaments	**Ruta**, Rhus tox
Sunburn	Dry, hot, red, throbbing, painful	Belladonna
	Blistering	Cantharis
Sunstroke	With fever and headache	Belladonna
	Shock and fear	Aconite
Whiplash	For injury and shock	Arnica
	Shooting nerve pain	Hypericum
	Injuries to ligaments or tendons	Ruta

ACUTE ILLNESS AND OTHER COMPLAINTS WHICH CAN BE TREATED THERAPEUTICALLY

Complaint	Symptoms	Remedies to consider
Boils	Small but sore	Arnica
	Hot and throbbing	Belladonna
	Slow healing	Silica

Complaint	Symptoms	Remedies to consider
Chicken-pox	At first onset with fever and restlessness	Aconite
	High fever and red face	Belladonna
	Clingy, weepy child, no thirst	Pulsatilla
	Worse at night, restless, chilly and **very itchy**	Rhus tox
Chillblains	Hot and itchy, worse heat	Pulsatilla
	Dark red inflammation, worse cold and damp	Rhus tox
Colds	Early stages, sneezing, thin burning watery discharge, chilliness	Aconite
	Heavy feeling, 'flu like aching, thirstless	Gelsemium
	Sneezing, goes to chest, burning headache, better for cool air	Bryonia
	Discharge profuse yellowish or pale green, thirstless	Pulsatilla
	Sneezing with nose dripping like a tap, clear discharge	Natrum mur
Cold sores	On lips	Rhus Tox, Sepia,
	Brought on by sun	**Natrum mur**
Colic	Abdomen distended, pains are cutting (cause children to toss about in agony), **inconsolable**, angry	Chamomilla
	Violent pain in spasms, **better for bending double, hard pressure**, warmth and lying on stomach	Colocynth
	Spasms of **cramp better for warmth** and pressure	Mag phos
Coughs & Croup	Dry, short cough starts suddenly, especially after windy, cold, dry weather	Aconite
	Dry cough with headache	

Complaint	Symptoms	Remedies to consider
Coughs & Croup (cont.)	and stitching pain in chest, worse movement	Bryonia
	Cough dry at night, loose **(yellowish green phlegm)** in the morning, feels sorry for self	Pulsatilla
	With ropey, **stringy green mucous**, worse in morning	Kali bich
	Chest rattles but no phlegm brought up, wants to be wrapped up, child may cry before coughing	Hepar sulph
	Hoarse, hollow barking cough sounds like a saw	Spongia
Cystitis	Cutting, burning pain before/during/after urination, urine passes drop by drop	Cantharis
	Stinging, burning sharp pain when passing few drops of hot urine	Apis
	During honeymoon and generally when worse after sex	Staphisagria
Dental visits	Fear and anxiety or panic	Aconite
	Shakiness and anxiety causing desire to pass stool or urine	Gelsemium
	Before fillings or extractions, for shock, bruising or hemorrhage	Arnica (one before and one after)
	After injections and for shooting nerve pains	Hypercium
	After mercury fillings when flu/cold symptoms follow	Merc viv
	For after effects from anaesthetic e.g. vomiting	Phosphorus
Diarrhoea	From fright	Aconite
	Caused by excitement or worrying about a forthcoming event	Arg nit

Complaint	Symptoms	Remedies to consider
	With vomiting caused by food poisoning	Arsenicum
	With colic (e.g. in babies), cramping, griping pains, better pressure and bending double	Colocynth
	Caused by anticipatory anxiety, may be trembling	Gelsemium
	Drives from bed in the morning	Sulphur
Earache	Starts suddenly after cold, dry winds, maybe fearful	Aconite
	Throbbing pain, causing child to cry out in sleep, high fever	Belladonna
	Inconsolable from pain, child wants to be carried, may accompany teething	Chamomilla
	Worse evening and night, cattarh blocking Eustachian tube tearful, whiny wants lots of comforting	Pulsatilla
	Perforated eardrum or blocked with hard wax, deafness from cattarh, timid, shy children	Silica
	Spasmodic shooting pain, better for warmth/pressure	Mag phos[1]
Examination nerves	Anticipation and dread with diarrhoea, trembling or paralysis	Gelsemium
	Nervous and hurried, diarrhoea, the 'what if' remedy	Arg nit

---

[1] Mag Phos is often called the homeopathic 'aspirin' because it is so good at easing pain. It works brilliantly for any complaint where the pains are sudden, shooting, darting or stabbing e.g. earache, stomach cramps/colic, period pains which are better from the onset of the flow, sciatica, teething, toothache, spasmodic cramps and neuralgia and when pains are better from warmth, pressure and bending double. This remedy works best when dissolved in warm water and sipped slowly.

Complaint	Symptoms	Remedies to consider
Frozen shoulder	Sore, bruised and **stiff** with tearing, shooting, stitching pains; better for heat and hot bath; **worse** at night, worse **resting** (too uncomfortable)	Rhus tox
	Bruised, sore, aching with restlessness; **better** for warmth, motion and **rubbing**; worse for damp, wet and wind	Ruta
Hangovers	Too much food/drink, irritability, headache and nausea	Nux vom
Headaches	Sudden onset, from chill, shock or fright	Aconite
	From excitement or over exertion; **throbbing pain**, during period, eyes sensitive to light	Belladonna
	Pain in forehead, may extend to the neck and shoulders, **worse for movement** and dry cough	Bryonia
	Heavy **dull ache**, begins in neck, sensation of a tight band around the head, from stress or apprehension	Gelsemium
	From too much to eat or drink, with nausea	Nux vom
	Gastric headaches, worse ices	Pulsatilla
Inoculations	Before to reduce local reaction, or after for shooting pains	Hypericum
	For puncture wound	Ledum
	Before during and after for exhaustion	Arnica
Measles	For sudden onset with fever and dry cough, sneezing,	

Complaint	Symptoms	Remedies to consider
	sore eyes, runny nose and fear or anxiety	Aconite
	Bright red rash with burning hot skin, throbbing headache with dilated pupils	Belladonna
	Slow onset, harsh, dry cough, worse movement (child may scream), thirsty; rash late to develop or incomplete	Bryonia
	Eyes stream and itch with burning tears, worse for light; rash around eyes, runny nose	Euphrasia
	Slow onset with shuddering chills up and down the spine; with drowsiness, headache, heaviness of limbs and droopy eyelids	Gelsemium
	Eyes itch and run, catarrh, loose cough by day (dry at night); thirstless, child tearful and clingy, may be earache	Pulsatilla
	Very itchy purple rash which is slow to develop; useful for symptoms which fail to clear up when the disease has run its course	Sulphur
Menstrual problems	Nausea before/during period, early period with passage of clots or bright red blood	Ipecac
	Cramping **pain**, better for bending double	**Mag phos**
	Pain with nausea and faintness	Nux vom
	Scanty periods with pain in lower back; pain ceases when flow starts	Pulsatilla
	Period late, scanty and irregular or early and	

Complaint	Symptoms	Remedies to consider
Menstrual problems (cont.)	profuse; with bearing down sensation	Sepia
Morning sickness	**Nausea**, belching, retching with pale face; worse after eating and smell of food	**Ipecac**
	Nausea, flatulence, retching, vomiting, feels faint; worse after eating, worse morning	Nux vom
	Worse thinking about food; empty, sinking feeling in the stomach, vomiting; temporarily better for eating	Sepia
Mouth ulcers	Ulcers, mouth/tongue, increased saliva/bad breath	Merc viv
Mumps	Useful at onset, restlessness, fever and anxiety	Aconite
	Bright red face, swelling worse on right side, very thirsty, sensitive to light, noise and draughts; delirious	Belladonna
	For problems with breasts, ovaries or testes; where patient feels chilly but wants fresh air	Carbo veg
	With smelly sweat/breath	Merc viv
	Glands very hard, pain shoots into ears when swallowing	Phytolacca
	Breasts, ovaries or testes affected, children are clingy and whining	Pulsatilla
	Dark red swelling, worse on the left side, maybe cold sores on lips	Rhus tox
Nails	Nails which split or have white spots; use 6c potency three times daily; **do not**	

Complaint	Symptoms	Remedies to consider
Nails (cont.)	**use if history of Tuberculosis or if patient has any form of implants/ pacemaker etc.**	Silca
Nausea	Diarrhoea and vomiting from **food poisoning**; anxious, chilly and restless	Arsenicum
	Bitter vomiting after eating, worse for movement	Bryonia
	Nausea not better for vomiting, with clean red tongue	Ipecac
	After **too much alcohol** or rich food	**Nux vom**
	Vomiting immediately food or drink is warmed in stomach; **post-operative vomiting**; burning in throat/ bowels, better for ice cold food or drink; stomach painful from touch	Phosphorus
	Vomiting from fatty, rich food; stomach feels heavy; no thirst	Pulsatilla
Nosebleeds	When period overdue or in the morning relieving a headache	Bryonia
Pre-Menstrual Tension	Weepy, oversensitive, changeable moods, irregular periods	Pulsatilla
	Sad/depressed with scanty periods, tiredness	Sepia
	For other symptoms see your homeopath	
Sadness	Sadness with sighing; after bereavement; maybe hysterical	Ignatia
	Gloomy, depressed; keeps feelings inside, won't cry except when alone	Natrum mur

Complaint	Symptoms	Remedies to consider
Sadness (cont.)	Weepy, better for company and consolation, changeable moods.	Pulsatilla
Scarlet Fever	**Swollen** stinging sore throat, skin mottled, face **puffy** with red and white blotches drowsy; worse warm room	Apis
	Number one remedy, with hot bright red face, red eyes, pupils dilated, throbbing headache, thirsty	**Belladonna**
	Ulcerated throat with painful tonsils	Lachesis
	Rash slow to appear with small blisters, sleepy but restless, better from warmth, worse at night, may be delirious	Rhus tox
Sciatica	Number one remedy, dull stitching pain starting in hip and shooting down to back of thigh, knee or foot	**Colocynth**
	Lightening pains, worse right side, better for warmth	Mag phos
	Tearing pain in thighs after exposure to cold/wet, or after muscular exertion/ overstraining, worse in bed at rest, during night; **numbness, stiffness;** extreme pain on first movement eases after walking a little	Rhus tox
	Pain extends from back to hips and thighs, better pressure and lying on back, worse lying down at night; restless, bruised aching pain; despairing with weariness and weakness	Ruta

Complaint	Symptoms	Remedies to consider
Sciatica (cont.)	Sciatica alternating with cough	Staphysagria
Shingles	Large blisters which sting and burn; red and puffy; better for cold applications, worse warmth and touch; patient restless	Apis
	Violent burning pain better for hot, dry applications, patient may be anxious	Arsenicum
	Intolerable burning and itching which stays after the rash has gone; **worse night** and for warmth and touch	Mezereum
	Dry, hot, burning, itching, skin sensitive to cold air; small blisters; tearing shooting pains; patient anxious and despondent	Rhus tox
	Stinging, smarting pain prior to attack of shingles; worse touch, worse anger; itching changes place after scratching	Staphysagria
Sore throats	Sudden acute inflammation dry, red, burning throat	Aconite
	Very swollen with stinging, burning pains; worse warm drinks, better cold drinks	Apis
	Dry, red, hot throat with swollen tonsils/glands; may have throbbing headache	Belladonna
	Mouth and throat dry, thirsty; worse movement	Bryonia
	Slow onset sore throat with flu type aching and weakness	Gelsemium
	Swelling of tonsils/neck glands; pain in throat which extends to ears on swallowing, as if fish-bone is stuck	Hepar sulph

Complaint	Symptoms	Remedies to consider
Sore throats (cont.)	Sore throat starts on the left but may move to the right; worse swallowing saliva, liquids, especially hot drinks, pain to ear	Lachesis
	Throat dark red or bluish red; swollen tonsils/uvula; **pain at root of tongue** and shooting to ears on swallowing	Phytolacca
Stiff neck	From cold wind or draught	Aconite
	Stiffness and pain, worse for movement	Bryonia
Stye	Lid swollen, puffy, red; stinging pain worse for heat, better cold application	Apis
	Itching eye with sticky yellow discharge	Pulsatilla
	Sty which develops into hard lump, swollen tear duct	Silica
	Recurring styes especially with suppressed anger	Staphysagria
Teething	**Cross/angry** with pain which is worse for hot drinks and better for cold; one cheek red the other pale, may have colic and diarrhoea	Chamomilla
	Teething pain better hot drinks and pressure, worse cold	Mag phos
Thrush	Discharge thick creamy or watery or yellow/green	Pulsatilla
	Lumpy and offensive yellow green discharge	Sepia
Travel sickness	Difficult to vomit but better after	Nux Vom
	Worse for fresh air	Petroleum
	Better for fresh air, worse opening eyes	Tabac

Complaint	Symptoms	Remedies to consider
Vomiting	With diarrhoea, from **food poisoning**, anxious and restless	Arsenicum
	Bitter vomiting after food or drink; worse movement	Bryonia
	Constant nausea, not better from vomiting; tongue clean or bright red	Ipecac
	Nausea after too much to eat or drink; better if could vomit, may be worse mornings	Nux vom
	Vomits immediately food or drinks warm up in the stomach; belching; post operative vomiting	Phosphorus
	Stomach feels heavy, worse after fatty food/ice cream/fruit; flatulence; thirstless	Pulsatilla
Warts	Crops of warts	Thuja
	On arms, hands, eyelids and face; many very small warts	Causticum
Whooping cough	General treatment; Cough triggered by movement, food or drink; coughing leads to vomiting; better in cool open air and for pressure; very thirsty	Pertussin
		Bryonia
	Worse from midnight until three or four in the morning; worse lying down; tickling dry throat; cough until vomit	Drosera
	Typical cough, plus bleeding from nose or mouth; rattling mucous in the chest, nausea, vomiting, clean tongue; convulsions	Ipecac

8
•••••

A Simple Materia Medica

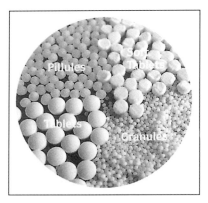

TYPICAL PREPARATIONS
FOR REMEDIES
Pillules, soft tablets, tablets, granules

T his chapter provides a simple check-list of remedies to see which one covers a particular complaint and, more especially, whether it is indicated by one or more of the other factors listed. If you match the complaint and recognize some of the other signs given, then that remedy is likely to be the most effective one.

• **ACONITE**

Top remedy for stopping colds from developing

A n excellent remedy for the first signs of colds, *fevers and inflammations*. If this remedy is taken early enough, it can prevent the complaint from developing fully. It is suited to symptoms that develop suddenly. There may be a lot of *sneezing* with either a dry or a very runny nose. The *throat* is likely to be very red and inflamed with burning and dryness. The patient may have a high temperature. If there is a cough, it may be a constant *short dry cough* with tightness of the chest but little wheezing or expectoration. Possible causes are exposure to cold, dry winds, fright or shock. The patient may show signs of restlessness, anxiety and fear, and in extreme cases may be afraid that they will die. Complaints which come on suddenly in the night.

Sleeplessness with restlessness and agitation. *Insomnia* in the aged. Sudden violent headaches, especially with restlessness, anguish, fever and fear. Sudden *earache*, with sensitivity to noise and music, which is unbearable. The beginning of *Influenza*. Thirst and restlessness are always present and there may be a cold sweat.

Use in the early stages of *measles*, also in high potency to remove foreign bodies from the eyes; and for bleeding and painful *haemorrhoids* that itch, particularly at night.

• APIS

This is the top remedy for stings and bites

T here is likely to be *swelling* with oedema, *puffiness and redness*. The pain will be burning or stinging. Symptoms are likely to be better for cold applications and worse for heat. The patient may be *thirstless*. This remedy can be useful where there is grief, fright, jealousy, rage, vexation or over-excitement.

• ARGENT NITRATE

Top remedy for a fear of flying and anxiety about travelling generally

A lso useful for *anticipatory anxiety* ('what if?'), often with digestive problems and diarrhoea or bloating, belching and flatulence. There may be a fear (of failing) when performing in public. Failure may occur as a result of rushing things. Fear of fainting. The patient is worse for eating sweets (diarrhoea) or being in crowded places. Pains may be splinter-like.

Conjunctivitis and other eye problems, which may alternate with digestive problems.

• ARNICA

Top remedy for accidents, shock and exhaustion

U sed for swelling and bruising, and soreness, especially to soft tissue or muscle. Give Arnica as soon as possible after injury and it will *promote healing*. Use in cases of shock, when the patient says 'I'm fine'. After head injuries, but watch for signs of concussion, and seek additional help if appropriate. Use before and after a trip to the dentist, especially for pain *after tooth extraction* and fillings. Use for shock and pain immediately after burns. Helpful for bruised pain in lower abdomen during periods, particularly if alternating with depression.

The patient is worse for being touched, motion, rest, damp and cold, but is better for lying down with their head low.

• ARSENICUM

Top remedy for food poisoning

U se for gastro-enteritis and stomach problems with diarrhoea, which are worse for iced water, ice cream, tobacco, or vinegar. The patient is likely to be chilly with great anxiety and restlessness. Or they may be completely prostrated. Pains are burning and the patient is generally better for warm applications and hot drinks.

This is a good remedy to take on holiday for vomiting and diarrhoea e.g. from food poisoning. Can be useful in cases where the patient feels burning hot and is anxious, perhaps with bad dreams or hallucinations (e.g. influenza), especially with a fear of death or great anxiety about their health.

• BELLADONNA

Top remedy for fevers

T *hrobbing pains*, and glassy eyes with dilated pupils are characteristic of this remedy.

Useful for sore, red throats and tonsillitis. The patient is dry and hot to touch, radiating heat. They may have a red face and experience hallucinations. There may also have been violent **headaches** with throbbing pains.

There may be a rapid pulse. A very useful remedy for **sunstroke**. In cases of **meningitis**, 'phone for an ambulance and give a dose of belladonna, every 10 minutes while waiting for it to arrive.

• BRYONIA

Top remedy for dry painful coughs and also headaches

H eadaches are bursting and splitting with nausea, and sometimes vertigo. There is often faintness on standing or sitting up . The patient is **worse from the slightest movement**. They are likely to be irritable and thirsty, with dry lips and mouth. Useful for **nosebleeds**. And also very useful for colds and coughs which start with sneezing and a runny nose and eyes. The patients eyes and body ache. The cold may go down to the patient's throat and larynx (with hoarseness) and then it may travel down into their lungs leading to bronchitis. A dry spasmodic cough shakes the whole body. There is very little expectoration. The patient is worse at night and on entering a warm room; also after eating and drinking.

• CALENDULA

Top remedy to assist the healing process

T he '*homeopathic antiseptic*' Used in cases of *cuts, burns and scalds*. Will help ruptured eardrums to heal properly. Use to assist healing following childbirth and tooth extraction. Calendula is very helpful *after surgery* when it can be given to promote the formation of healthy scar tissue.

• CANTHARIS

Top remedy for cystitis with burning and smarting pains before, during and after urination (especially where there is greater urgency to urinate)

T he onset of complaints is sudden and violent. Also a very useful remedy for the pain of burns. Patients are very thirsty, but worse for drinking, urination and touch. Use for blisters from burns and sunburn. This remedy can be useful for shingles and skin eruptions with large blisters. Better for warmth, rest and rubbing. Can be useful for nosebleeds.

• CARBO VEG

Top remedy for collapse, especially when a patient is unable to get enough oxygen

T he patient may be blue and have a cold sweat. Give this remedy immediately and seek help. Useful for extreme weakness and faintness, especially when a patient feels very cold but is a worse in a warm, stuffy room. The patient may desire stimulants such as coffee and acidic things. This remedy is excellent for very bad indigestion with bloating and incarcerated wind that is likely to cause explosive belching.

The patient will be better in cooler air, being fanned or after burping.

• CAUSTICUM

Top remedy for involuntary urination when sneezing, coughing or walking

A lso use for warts especially on the face, eyelids, nose and around the nails. Useful in burns, especially chemical. Other uses are for bed wetting, incessant tickly coughs (better for sipping cold drinks) and rheumatism. Complaints are worse on the right side and may be brought on by dry cold winds. Better for damp, rainy weather, being warm in bed.

• CHAMOMILLA

The top remedy for teething and colic in children

C omplaints accompanied by irritation or anger. The patient is inconsolable. Patients may be hot and sweaty (especially on the scalp). Also useful for toothache (worse for warm food or drink) and hard dry coughs (especially during sleep). One cheek may be flushed. Pain during menstruation and labour pains. The patient is worse from heat, anger and in the evening between a 9.00 pm and midnight, but will be better from warmth, wet weather and fasting.

• COLOCYNTHUS

This is an excellent remedy for colic and painful periods, with waves of pain

I t is especially helpful for pain which is cutting, stabbing, pinching and *cramping*. The patient is worse from emotions, especially anger. *Better from bending double, hard pressure*, heat, rest, and lying on the painful side.

• DROSERA

Top remedy for whooping cough

T he cough is a deep barking cough which takes the breath away. There may also be retching and vomiting. Also useful for asthma, bronchitis and measles. The patient will be worse lying down and after midnight. Better for pressure and in the open-air.

• EUPHRASIA

Top remedy for conjunctivitis and other eye disorders especially in measles

B urning eye secretions, with a bland nasal discharge. Eye strain from prolonged use of computer. The characteristic pain is burning and feeling sore.

• GELSEMIUM

Top remedy for influenza (and complaints remaining afterwards)

I t is especially helpful where the patient is very weak, weary, lethargic and dull. Also useful for pre-menstrual headaches, measles and *examination-type nerves and stage fright*, especially where there is diarrhoea from anxiety. The patient feels really heavy, and is reluctant to move. Complaints come on slowly over a few days.

The patient may be shaking, shivering or trembling and is usually thirstless (even during a fever). They appear to be 'dizzy, drowsy, droopy and dumb', and want to be left alone. They are likely to feel better from urination, sweating, shaking, shivering, and from alcohol. Vision may be blurred, with eyes feeling droopy/heavy and a headache travelling from the back of the head (hammering pain) over the top and resting above the eyes. The patient will be worse from anticipation, cold, damp weather and the heat of the sun.

• HEPAR SULPH

Top remedy for painful septic wounds (often with a lot of puss) and abscesses

D ischarges can smell bad, like rotting cheese. Pain the patient is extremely sensitive to cold air and draughts. Use also for *croupy, barking coughs* (worse for cold drinks) with rattling loose phlegm which is difficult to bring up; catarrh, cold sores, earache, *glandular swelling*, *tonsillitis* and quinsy (with pain extending into the ears on swallowing), toothache and styes. Pains in all complaints tend to be stitching and splinter like. The patient is likely to be better for heat, moist weather and lying in a warm bed. Worse for touch, cold dry air and cold drinks. They are generally over-sensitive to pain and aggravated by touch. Mentally and emotionally they are likely to be cross, *irritable* and easily upset when sick. Can be used to expel *splinters*.

• HYPERICUM

Top remedy for injury to parts rich in nerves

C *rushing injuries* such as when fingers are squashed in doors, or something has been dropped on the toes Also used for *injuries to the coccyx* (base of spine) and injuries from sharp objects; and in cases of laceration. In these type of injuries give Hypericum and wash the wound very thoroughly under cold running water to reduce the possible risk of tetanus. Also useful after animal or insect *bites*.

Pains are intense, and extend along the path of the nerve. Can help with pain after surgery or dental work. Other uses include frostbite, forceps delivery, vaccination and after a spinal tap (particularly where health problems follow).

The patient may be in a state of shock and worse for touch. Pain may be better for rubbing. After an accident, give Arnica for shock, followed by Hypericum for nerve pain.

Use for shooting pains in neck, back and down the legs. Take Arnica followed by Hypericum prior to and after root canal work. This remedy is also useful after injuries to the head with severe pain. It is the number one remedy for **whiplash injuries** (e.g. after a car accident).

• IPECAC

Top remedy for morning sickness and whooping cough

S uffocating cough with rattling of mucous, but unable to bring it up. Nausea and vomiting (including mucous), worse mornings; with a clean tongue (if the tongue is dirty white or yellow then consider Pulsatilla). Headaches (both sides of head) with nausea. The patient can be very pale or may have a bluish red face. Feels worse lying down, for motion, after overeating, eating rich food, vomiting, tobacco; and may be oversensitive to heat and cold. They are better in the open air, for cold drinks and for rest.

• KALI BICH

Top remedy for colds and sinus problems particularly with greenish coloured mucus Discharges are characteristically greenlyellow, thick and stringy and may smell

• LACHESIS

Use for sore throats and tonsillitis which are worse
for swallowing liquids and saliva

A lso good for *headaches*, with waves of pain; especially from the sun, and on awakening. Sore throats are likely to be dry and swollen inside and out, and made worse by hot drinks. Both the throat and tonsils can appear livid and *purplish* and *pains may extend to the ear*. Toothache with pain extending into the ear.

All complaints tend to *start on the left and move to the right* and come on during (or are worse after) sleep. The patient may have a *very pale face*, sometimes with red cheeks. They are generally worse on the left side, *worse for* a warm bath, hot drinks, closing their eyes, and especially for pressure or *constriction* of any sort.

• MAG PHOS

Top remedy for pain. 'The homeopathic aspirin'

E arache, headaches, toothache and menstrual pain. Pains are cramping or shooting; worse for cold and touch, but better for heat and firm pressure. Useful for neuralgia of the face and head. This remedy works extremely well when dissolved in warm water and sipped.

• MERC VIV

Top remedy for mouth ulcers

A lso useful for *sore throats, boils, abscesses, headaches, joint pains, thrush, toothache, cystitis and ear infections*. Discharges usually smell offensive. Patients may have excessive saliva, but are likely to be very thirsty.

The patient will be very sensitive to heat and cold, preferring moderate temperatures. They are usually worse at night, in warm damp weather, lying on their right side, perspiring, and it in a warm room or warm bed.

• MEZERIUM

Top remedy for cradle cap

U se for intensely itchy eczema. The patient is generally worse for cold damp air, touch, and at night until midnight. They may be better for being in the open air.

• NATRUM MUR

Top remedy for cold sores on the lips

A lso good for colds with a clear watery nasal discharge, coughs with bursting headaches, sunstroke and clear blistery spots. Patients may suffer from a split in the centre of their lower lip. Complaints are worse during the morning, by the sea, from the sun and in cold weather. They generally feel better in the open air.

• NUX VOMICA

Top remedy for hangovers

U se for headaches, ***indigestion***, ***stomach upsets*** (feels as if there is a stone in the stomach), nausea and vomiting; especially where the patient has had too much to eat or drink. They may be ***irritable*** (or angry), tense (perhaps with palpitations) and oversensitive. Other possible symptoms include insomnia, constipation and piles. Useful for ***workaholics*** who thrive on the stimulants and relaxants (coffee/alcohol/cigarettes etc.). High blood pressure could also be present. The patient is ***worse in the morning***, worse for drafts, lack of sleep, alcohol, touch, light and noise. They may be better for rest, moist air, milk, fats and hot drinks.

• PHOSPHORUS

Top remedy for hepatitis and jaundice

U seful in tight, dry coughs, laryngitis and nausea during pregnancy. This remedy can help with the ***after effects of anaesthetics***; and when patients ***bleed profusely or haemorrhage*** after cuts, teeth extraction or surgery. The patient is likely to be chilly and may crave ice-cream and be thirsty for cold drinks (although these can sometimes lead to vomiting). There may be anxiety or fears present. They are likely to be worse for lying on their left side, missing a meal, and for strong emotions, odours and anaesthetics (particularly gas). Patients requiring phosphorus are generally better for eating and sleeping (even a short nap).

• PULSATILLA

> ### *Top remedy for childhood earaches and complaints with yellow/greenish, thick catarrh*

A lso consider for mumps, measles, *varicose veins*, hay fever, chilblains and mastitis. Children are *clingy and whiny*, needing lots of cuddles and sympathy. Patients may be *tearful*, moody and crave company. They are often *thirstless* and keen to have windows and doors open, in order to get plenty of fresh air.

Symptoms are often very changeable, but the patient invariably feels better for consolation. They are worse in stuffy rooms and around twilight (bedtime)!

• RHUS TOX

> ### *Top remedy for joints, muscle aches, sprains and strains, rheumatism and shingles*

V ery useful for mumps, chicken-pox and nettle rash.

Stiffness and aches are *worse on first movement*, but soon become better for continued movement (although may get worse again after a while). Patients may be rather sad and weepy for no particular reason. They are usually very restless, chilly, and very much worse for cold and damp weather, but better for a warm bath.

● **RUTA**

Top remedy for over stretching tendons and ligaments, and for problems with the surface of bones (periosteum)

P atients may be a little restless and irritable. The pains are generally worse when resting and better for movement. Rheumatic pains are aggravated by cold, damp weather. Joints feel as if they could give way. The most affected parts are the **ankles, wrists, knees** and **shins**. Injuries very often occur from over use of joints e.g. tennis elbow and repetitive strain injuries. Very useful remedy to deal with **lameness** following an injury.

● **SEPIA**

Useful for stretch marks after pregnancy and for morning sickness

A lso helpful for constipation, hot flushes at menopause, painful periods, PMT and prolapsed womb. Patients are often worse for the smell, sight and the thought of food. They commonly feel a dragging-down sensation . Usually they will be better for vigorous exercise such as dancing, horse riding, or fairground rides. They may have a strong aversion to tobacco smoke and are often quite irritable.

● **SILICA**

Top remedy for expelling splinters etc.

T his remedy will expel foreign bodies – so beware if you have had any implants (e.g.

metal pins/ pacemaker etc.)! Will improve the growth and quality of the hair and nails (e.g. if brittle and breaking). Useful for adhesions (when several different layers of tissue stick together) after operations. Helps stop constipation, especially when the stool slips back; and is useful for headaches (usually start at the back of the head but may spread forwards and settle over the eyes) with constipation. Silica can also be used to deal with ill effects after vaccination, for recurrent quinsy and throaty colds with swollen glands.

• STAPHYSAGRIA

Top remedy for styes

S taphysagria is a good remedy to use for sore throats, with stitching pains running to the ears (especially left) on swallowing. Very often extremely helpful for pain following cuts/surgery, especially to the reproductive organs (*episiotomy* etc.), bladder, abdomen and anus. Other uses are to help prevent mosquito bites, discourage head lice, for spongy bleeding gums, for shingles, and morning sickness, *feeling of violation*; and for colic after anger especially in children with a swollen abdomen and flatulence (hot).

Use for stupefying headaches (which may feel a bit better for yawning). The pain can be so great that the patient wants to bang their head against a wall. The sensation is of a ball of lead in the forehead. Helps to combat *nausea after operations*.

Very effective for dealing with *cystitis/irritable bladder* especially after frequent intercourse: also the bladder may feel as if it will not empty properly (as if under pressure) after (frequent) urging to urinate. There may be a sensation as if a drop of urine were rolling continuously along the channel, a burning feeling (when not urinating), or splinter-like pain after urination.

Symptoms are generally worse for anger, grief, indignation, humiliation and touch; especially when feelings have been suppressed. The patient is often better for warmth and rest.

• SULPHUR

Useful for the itchy purple rash of measles; and when measles or other acute diseases have more or less run their course, but failed to clear up completely

T he remedy can also be very effective in dealing with *diarrhoea* that drives the patient out of bed in the morning. The patient is hot; any pains may be of a burning nature. Anyone needing this remedy is likely to be worse around 11am, for warmth in bed, for washing and bathing. They may be better in dry warm weather, lying on their right side and drawing up their limbs.

9 ·····

Going to the Homeopath

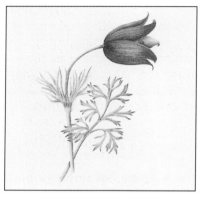

WIND OR PASQUE FLOWER
Source of the homeopathic remedy
Pulsatilla nigricans

WHEN TO SEEK PROFESSIONAL HELP

Most people who have uncomfortable or unpleasant symptoms, simply want to get relief from those symptoms. This in itself is not healing, because symptoms are our alarm call that something is wrong at a deeper level. Switch off your burglar alarm if it keeps going off in the night and you might sleep comfortably for a few hours; but watch out in the morning when you finally face up to what was causing the inconvenience! Ignoring early warnings about your health is at best unfair to yourself, and at worst putting your health (potentially) at serious risk.

As we noted earlier, it is quite possible to stop symptoms without healing taking place. In fact, merely stopping the body (e.g. using self-treatment / drugs or surgery) from giving us the warning signs that something is wrong, can mean that we avoid or delay true healing. This can be dangerous as it allows our health to degenerate, while on the surface we appear OK. Eventually, we will get another more serious warning to take action, but by then we are likely to be a lot sicker.

The first sign that something is wrong is often simply that we notice that our body has changed the way that it functions, for longer than a few days at a time (as may be the case in acute illnesses), or repeatedly. This is a good time to arrange a visit to a professional homeopath. The difficulty is that these changes may have occurred gradually over a period of months or even years. So the first thing we need to ensure, is that we are aware of our mental or emotional and physical well-being, and secondly that we do not ignore the warning signs, put up with them or accept them as inevitable. Take action now. Find a homeopath who can support your choice to live in the best health possible for you.

Ideally, you will act even before functional changes become apparent. Health does not just happen. Sickness does, unless we continually act to live in health (by nurturing our body/mind and spirit). 'Constitutional' homeopathic treatment from a professional homeopath can help you prevent even functional disease from occurring. The aim in this case being to maintain your optimum health rather than restore it when you have lost it.

Sadly, too, many people fall into a third category. Symptomatic relief through drugs or surgery is used for as long as possible. After a number of years chronic health problems are so bad that in desperation, patients finally decide enough is enough and seek an alternative to the treatments which have failed to maintain their health (and in many cases contributed to additional health problems) over the years.

Why the reluctance to choose healing rather than settle for symptomatic relief? Basically, healing involves agreeing to change whatever it is in our lives that has led to a decline in our health. It is foolish to think that by living in exactly the same way that led to our sickness we can improve our health.

But the hardest thing for any of us to do is change, even if our life depends upon it. If you doubt that, then you will be surprised at the mother who when told that her child's healing from cancer may be assisted by cutting out sugar in the form of sweets, replied that under no circumstances would she deprive her of sweets. On another occasion, a lady suffering cancer for a second time, decided against having homeopathic constitutional treatment when she was advised to reduce or give up her daily intake of coffee. And these are physical habits. How much more difficult to change negative mental or emotional patterns?

HOW TO CHOOSE A HOMEOPATH

J ust as each patient is unique so each homeopath is an individual. However, if you want to ensure that your chosen homeopath is of a good standard, then the easiest way is to check that they belong to one of the recognized professional associations with a published code of ethics by which they will have agreed to abide. In order to gain membership they have had to gain appropriate qualifications and satisfy other entry requirements. (*See Appendix.*)

Your homeopath is going to be your main ally in helping you to bring about the necessary changes for healing to take place. You need to find one to whom you can talk freely and honestly, in order that they can decide on the most appropriate treatment. Personal recommendations from family or friends are often useful, but do also check out the practitioner's qualifications and whether they are registered with the appropriate professional organization.

Some homeopaths offer short sessions free of charge, when you can meet them and ask questions before committing to treatment. This can be particularly useful, in that you will be able to get a feeling for whether or not you will be able to work with her/him. It helps when talking to your practitioner, if you feel that you are in a safe non-judgemental place. In this way you will feel able to freely and openly discuss any and all of your symptoms, as well as your hopes and fears.

Having opted for homeopathic treatment, another question to ask yourself is, do you want a fully-trained and experienced homeopath to treat you, or would you settle for an allopathic doctor who may have had shorter training or less experience in homeopathy? There are some practitioners who are fully qualified in both disciplines; however, because the two forms of medicine use such different models of treatment, this is not very common. It is difficult to have a foot in both camps, although some practitioners who are fully qualified homeopaths and allopaths seem to be able to switch hats appropriately and have a great deal of training and experience from both schools to offer. Just be clear where your practitioner is coming from, and choose what you feel comfortable with.

To complicate matters further, homeopaths can be separated into those who follow the classical school of homeopathy (where high potencies of remedies are prescribed in single doses infrequently) and those who use a variety of approaches when they prescribe, based on the differing needs of their patients. In many ways homeopaths are more like family doctors used to be. You get to know each other during the healing process and it is important that there is mutual respect. Homeopaths do not claim to be specialists (although they may well have great experience and a high reputation for success with a particular disease). By considering the whole individual they are open to seeing the real cause of an individuals dis-ease wherever that may be found. However, if it is appropriate to obtain an allopathic diagnosis then this will be suggested.

WHAT IS HOMEOPATHIC TREATMENT LIKE?

Many first-time patients are very pleasantly surprised at the depth of the initial consultation. Typically this will last for between an hour and an hour-and-a-half. Some patients have never before experienced this degree of attentiveness from any other human being, and if appropriate this can lead to them sharing things that they have never spoken of to anyone. This in itself can be a very powerful start to the healing process. One patient commented during her second visit: 'I felt totally unburdened as I walked down the street after the first consultation.' And that was before she had received any treatment!

Your homeopath is there to support you mentally, emotionally and physically in your journey to health. In theory, all she/he has to do is spend an hour or so chatting to you, to find out your particular symptoms, and then find the remedy or remedies that match those symptoms. However, people are often very unused to talking openly about their physical problems, let alone mental or emotional issues. A visit to the homeopath should represent a safe, confidential and non-judgemental space where you can drop any mask that you wear for the world, and get in touch with the real you. This in itself is such a release for many people, that it is a very powerful stage in the healing process, even before any remedies are taken.

THE QUESTIONNAIRE

B efore your first appointment, you may be asked to complete a questionnaire giving details of your own medical history, and that of your family. This is so that your homeopath can see how other health issues may have contributed to your current problems, and what patterns of suscep- tibility to particular illnesses (miasms) you may have inherited from your parents, grandparents etc. You are also likely to be asked about any medication that you are taking, as well as any supplements. The questionnaire will also ask you for brief details of the health issue or issues which you want to consult the homeopath about. Although many of us do not enjoy filling in questionnaires, it does save valuable time during the first consultation, which can then be spent gaining information in greater detail and building a rapport between practitioner and patient.

One of the things which often surprises people on their first visit to a homoeopath is the amount of detail they require. This applies not only to your main complaint, but also to your lifestyle, bodily functions, food likes and dislikes, fears and phobias. You may also be asked about your preferences with regard to the weather and your location (e.g. in fresh mountain air or by the sea). All of this information can to be helpful in the process of finding the best remedies for you as an individual. The more open, honest and frank that you can be from the start, then the more quickly and thoroughly your homeopath is likely to be able to help you.

For many of us this is a new experience. In attempting to describe our symptoms accurately we are often hearing and starting to understand consciously for the first time exactly what our body is trying to tell us. This could be seen as the second step towards healing. In order to answer the homeopath's questions, we need to consider what makes us feel better or worse. When do we feel better or worse? Exactly how do we feel when we are upset. What sort of pain are we experiencing? Is it cutting, aching, throbbing, stabbing, burning etc.? What was happening in our life in the weeks, months or even the years before we became ill, which could have triggered our current condition. Often we know this at a subconscious level, but sometimes it is only when speaking out loud, that we acknowledge it and recognize our need to change. Step three is when we commit to the changes necessary to restore balance and health to our lives. The remedies are carefully selected to instigate or assist and support this healing process.

You will need to return for a follow-up visit to monitor your progress, and in order to decide if further remedies are required. Follow-up visits are shorter than the first one, usually lasting up to half an hour. How soon you return to see your homeopath, will depend on the following factors. The nature of your illness, the method of homeopathy used, and what you feel to be appropriate. It could be as little as a week (less for very severe or acute complaints) or as long as a couple of months or more. My own preference is to see patients fairly soon after their first experience of homeopathic remedies, in order to assess how well they are responding, and to answer any questions that may have arisen during the healing process. Your homeopath has training and experience in the variety of ways in which individuals can respond to treatment, as well as the effects each of the different remedies has.

If you have any questions, or there are changes in your condition which give rise to concern, it is important to discuss these with your homeopath in the first instance, rather than someone untrained in the science and art of homeopathy. Someone with no knowledge of the effect of homeopathic remedies on an individual, would be likely to misinterpret the signs. This could lead to incorrect diagnosis and inappropriate treatment as well as unnecessary anxiety for the patient. However, if you are unable to contact your homeopath immediately and you feel that the problem is urgent, then you should discuss it with a qualified medical practitioner without delay.

WHAT CAN I EXPECT TO HAPPEN?

Y ou can expect the healing process to begin. This does not always mean the symptoms will stop immediately. Remember that symptoms are the body's attempt to heal itself. Sometimes, in support of the healing process, the remedy will promote appropriate symptoms. For example, a discharge may temporarily become more profuse as the remedy helps the body to throw out mucus or other fluids in order to resolve the problem. This is why people often ask 'will I get worse before I get better?' There is no absolute answer to this question, other than to say that a temporary increase in the intensity of symptoms may occur before an improvement follows.

Everyone is different, and therefore everyone can expect to react slightly differently even to the same homeopathic remedy. Usually, if a remedy is not able to bring about a healing response, then it will do nothing at all and a new remedy will be selected. When the appropriate remedy is given then healing occurs from the inside and out, and moves from important organs to less important organs. For example, a child with asthma, who had previously suffered from eczema, would experience an improvement in the asthma although the eczema may return before the patient is finally healed. Remember, healing occurs in reverse order to which the symptoms originally appeared (direction of cure).

This return of old symptoms is a very good sign that healing is taking place. For this reason it is important that your homeopath monitors your treatment and prescribes any new remedies that are required to continue the direction of cure. If allopathic treatment is sought for symptoms occurring during this process, then healing is likely to be halted, and the suppression of symptoms may reverse the direction of cure, driving the disease deeper once again. If you have any doubts as to whether your reaction to a particular remedy is part of your healing process, then contact your homeopath who will be able to reassure you, or vary your treatment appropriately.

Homeopathy is much more than an instant cure. Rather it is a system of medicine, which over a period of time will support you in your attempt to become and stay as healthy as you possibly can. If this is what you seek then good luck. Homeopathy will serve you well.

10
●●●●●

Homeopathy and Prescribed Drugs

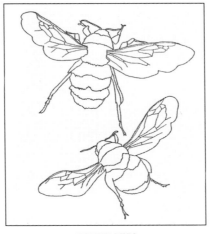

HONEY BEES
Source of the homeopathic remedy
apis

I t is important to remember that you are responsible for any drugs that you take. Yes, your doctor may have prescribed them for you and she/he is responsible for that prescription. But if you continue to take those drugs when you are aware that they are giving you serious side-effects, then you are the one who is responsible for the fact that you are experiencing such side-effects. Similarly, if you choose not to take drugs that have been prescribed for you, it is your decision and any consequences are your responsibility.

Homeopaths advise patients to discuss reducing or stopping prescribed drugs with their doctor. However, some doctor-patient relationships are so poor that the patient does not feel able to take on this responsibility. Doctors are very powerful figures, and for some patients, the thought of what they see as a challenge to their authority (and some doctors may feel challenged) is something that they cannot face.

This is not a healthy situation, as the patient has every right to an intelligent discussion on the pros and cons of treatment, and the final decision about her/his health. Any medical practitioner secure enough in his or her own professionalism, will not be offended by this. However, sadly, some practitioners abuse their power, and intimidate patients. It is up to patients to see this behaviour for what it is, and change their practitioner for one who is mature enough to work with them and support their right to make decisions about their health, even when he or she does not agree with them.

Patients often come with the express intention of reducing and eventually stopping orthodox drugs that are giving them unacceptable side-effects or which are addictive. Most doctors will respect the patient's choice and support this. However, a few may claim that only the drugs (and by implication only the doctor) can help the patient, and that homeopathic remedies interfere with the action of prescribed drugs (there is absolutely no evidence for this) and of course they have no effect anyway! On the contrary, the orthodox drugs may reduce the effect of the homeopathic remedies. Most homeopaths will discuss this fully with their patients, and use a variety of techniques to ensure that the remedies remain effective.

When a patient is receiving treatment from more than one source, it can sometimes make it more difficult to determine which treatment is doing what. However, with frank and honest discussion between patient and practitioner, and if necessary between practitioners, it is usually possible for all concerned to work together in respect of the patient's wishes.

The most important thing to remember, as previously noted, is that you are responsible for what happens to your body. Listen openly to advice and treatments offered, and make the decision that you are happy with, free from 'professional' intimidation. If you do decide to reduce prescribed drugs, then it is appropriate to discuss it with your doctor and try to enlist her/his support. For one thing it is courteous, and for another it can be dangerous to stop some drugs suddenly. I generally begin homeopathic treatment alongside orthodox drugs and then when the healing process is under way and the patient has started to feel the benefits, it is up to them to decide what they would like to do with regard to prescribed drugs.

It is very common for patients to seek homeopathic treatment, because they wish to avoid drugs with potentially harmful side-effects, or because they are experiencing unpleasant side-effects, or they are concerned about the dangers of addiction to prescribed drugs.

As well as using personal recommendations, check for membership of a professional organization, and try to choose a homeopath with whom you will be happy to work.

Appendix

• • • • •

How to Find a Homeopath

Use the websites listed below or contact the relevant organizations to request a list. Note that some organizations limit themselves to 'Classical' homeopaths only, and others include only those with allopathic medical qualifications.

UK

For a comprehensive online list of UK homeopathic practitioners by area see *The Institute of Homeopathy* website: *www.hominf.org.uk/list.htm* or you can use the UK Yellow Pages for 'homeopaths'.

A very useful website about homeopathy:
Website: *www.homeopathyhome.com*

The following organizations can help you locate a homeopathic practitioner in your area:

The Homeopathic Medical Association
6 Livingstone Road,
Gravesend,
Kent DA12 5DZ
Tel: 01474 560336
E-mail: *info@the-hma.org*

Society of Homeopaths
2 Artizan Road,
Northampton,
NN1 4HU
Tel: +44 (0)1604 621400
E-mail: *info@homeopathy-soh.org* or
societyofhomeopaths@btinternet.com (Has a register of qualified homeopaths)

The Faculty of Homeopathy & The Homeopathic Trust
15 Clerkenwell Close,
London EC1R 0AA
Faculty of Homeopathy Tel: +44 (0)207 566 7810
Homeopathic Trust Tel: +44 (0)207 566 7800 (Provides a list of qualified homeopaths with allopathic qualifications)

Association of Registered Homeopaths
Tel: 08700 736339

The British Hahnemann Society
2 Powis Place,
Great Ormond Street,
London WC1N 3HZ
Tel: +44 (0)207 837 3297

The British Homeopathic Association
27a Devonshire Street,
London W1N 1RJ
Tel: +44 (0)207 566 7800
E-mail: *info@trusthomeopathy.org* (Provides a list of qualified homeopaths with allopathic qualifications)

British Homeopathic Dental Association
2B Franklin Street,
Watford,
Herts WD1 1QD
Tel: 01923 233336

British Association of Homeopathic Veterinary Surgeons
Alternative Veterinary Medicine Centre
Chinham House,
Stanford-in-the-Vale,
Faringdon,
Oxon SN7 8NQ
Tel: 01367 710324

What some of the letters mean:
MHMA – Registered Member of the Homeopathic Medical Association
This means that the practitioner has passed a qualifying examination at a college approved by the Council of the Association or has proved his or her worthiness to practice to the satisfaction of the Council. They are bound by the Association's Code of Ethics and Practice and carry professional indemnity insurance. For further information contact:

The Homeopathic Medical Association
6 Livingstone Road,
Gravesend,
Kent DA12 5DZ
Tel: 01474 560336
E-mail: *info@the-hma.org*
Website: *http://www.the-hma.org*

RSHom – Registered Member of the Society of Homeopaths
This means that the practioner has qualified at a recognized college and then undergone the process of registration which involves at least a

year's practice, the presentation of cases and an inspection visit by the Society. RSHoms abide by the Society's Code of Ethics and Practice and are insured by the Society or have insurance approved by the Society. For further information contact:

Society of Homeopaths
2 Artizan Road,
Northampton,
NN1 4HU
Tel: +44 (0)1604 621400
E-mail: *societyofhomeopaths@btinternet.com*

MIH – Registered Member of the Institute of Homeopathy

This means that the practitioner has proved to the satisfaction of the Governing Council of the Institute that he or she has the knowledge, skills and commitment to practice homeopathy safely and effectively. Registered members agree to the Institute's Code of Ethical Practice and carry professional indemnity insurance. For further information contact:

The Institute of Homeopathy
23 Berkeley Road,
Bishopston,
Bristol BS7 8HF
Tel: 0117 944 5147
E-mail: *institute@hominf.org.uk*
Website: *http://www.hominf.org.uk*

NORTH AMERICA

American Foundation for Homeopathy
1508 S. Garfield,
Alhambra,
CA 91801 USA

American Institute of Homeopathy
1585 Glencoc St,
Ste 44, Denver,
CO 80220-1338 USA

Homeopathic Medical Society of New Mexico
122 Dartmouth,
Albuquerque,
NM 87106 USA

Homeopathic Medical Society of the State of Pennsylvania
Henshaw Health Center,
10 Skyport Rd,
Mechanicsburg,
PA 17055 USA

International Foundation for Homeopathy
2366 Fastiake Avenue E,
Ste 301, Seattle,
WA 98102 USA

National Center for Homeopathy and the American Board of Homeotherapeutics
801 North Fairfax St,
Ste 306, Alexandria,
VA 22314 USA
Tel: (703) 548-7790
E-mail: *nchinfo@iqc.apc.org*

New York Homeopathic Medical Society
110-56 71st Avenue,
Ste 1-H, Forest Hills,
NY 113751 USA

Ohio State Homeopathic Medical Society
800 Compton Rd,
Ste 24, Cincinnati,
OH 45231 USA

Southern Homeopathic Medical Association
10418 Whitehead St,
Fairfax,
VA 22030 USA

American Homeopathic Pharmacists Association
P.O. Box 60167,
Los Angeles,
CA 900061 USA

Homeopathic Academy of Naturopathic Physicians
11231 SE Market St,
Portland,
OR 97216 USA

Homeopathic Nurses Association
3403-17th Avenue So.,
Minneapolis,
MN 55407 USA

National Board of Homeopathy in Dentistry Inc
P.O. Box 423.
Marengo,
IL 60152 USA

Chiropractic Academy of Homeopathy
2536 Stadium Drive,
Zephyrhills,
FL 33540 USA

USA Organizations
There a number of searchable online databases and lists now available to help you to locate a homeopathic practitioner in your area:

The NCH Directory of Practitioners (Searchable)
website: *http://homeopathic.org/NCHsearch.htm*

The NCH also provides a useful State by State *Resources* page

The HANP searchable database of Members and Practitioners
website: *http://www.healthy.net/HANP/HANPsearch.htm*

The CHC searchable database of certified Practitioners
website: *http://www.healthy.net/asp/templates/center.asp?centerid=53*

The following organizations can also help you locate a homeopathic physician in your area.

American Institute of Homeopathy
801 North Fairfax Street Suite 306
Alexandria VA 22314
Tel: 703 246-9501

Homeopathic Academy of Naturopathic Physicians
P.O. Box 12488
Portland, OR 97212
Tel: (503) 795-0579

The Chiropractic Academy of Homeopathy
6536 Stadium Drive,
Zephyrhills,
Florida 33540
Tel: (813) 782-2690
Fax: (813) 782-3275
E-mail: *DANdc1@aol.com*

The Arizona Homeopathic Medical Association
2525 West Greenway Road Suite 300
Phoenix, Arizona 85023
Tel: (602) 978-1722
Fax: (602) 942-3787

Connecticut Homeopathic Association
P.O. Box 1055,
Greens Farms, CT 06436
Tel: (203) 327 6525
E-mail: *cha@simile.org*

The Academy of Veterinary Homeopathy
751 N E 168th St. N. Miami,
FL 33162-2427 305-652-1590
E-mail: *avh@naturalholistc.com*

CANADA

Canadian Foundation for Honicopathic Research and Development
P.O. Box 8213,
Station F,
Edmonton,
Alberta, T61-I 4P1

Canadian Society of Homeopathy
87 Meadowlands Drive West,
Nepean, Ontario, 1420 2R9

Centre de Techniques Homeopathiques
7 Laurier Avenue East,
Montreal,
Quebec, H2T 1E4

International Academy of Homeopathy and the Toronto Homeopathic Clinic
3255 Yonge St,
Toronto,
Ontario, M4N 2L5

AUSTRALIA

Australian Homoepathic Association
PO Box 396,
Drunmoyne,
New South Wales,

Australia 2047
Tel: +61 2 9719 2793

Australian Institute of Homeopathy
21 Bulah Close,
Berdwra Heights,
NSW, Australia 2082

Institute of Classical Homeopathy
24 West Raven Drive,
Tawa, Wellington,
New Zealand

Australian Centre for Homeopathy
I Para Road,
Tanunda,
SA 5352 Australia

Australian Council for Homeopathy (Vic)
151 Union St,
Winsor. Vic 3181
Australia

Australian Homeopathic Association (NSW)
P.O. Box 122,
Roseville,
NSW 2069
Australia.

Australian Homeopathic Association (SA)
44 Colton Avenue,
Maghul,
SA 5072
Australia.

NEW ZEALAND

There is a database of registered homeopathic practitioners by area on the NZCH site *http://www.homeopathy.co.nz/*

There is also a very comprehensive listing of homeopathic resources in the New Zealand Yellow Pages. *http://tdl.tols.co.nz/all-categories/health/alternative-health/homeopathy/index.html*

FURTHER READING

Miranda Castro — *Complete Homeopathy Handbook: A Guide to Everyday Healthcare* St. Martin's Press, 1991

Andrew Lockie — *Complete Guide to Homeopathy: The Principles and Practice of Treatment* DK Publishing, 1995

George Vithoulkas — *The Science of Homeopathy* Grove/Atlantic Inc, 1995

Christopher E. Day — *Homeopathic Treatment of Small Animals: Principles and Practice* Beekman Publishers Inc., 1992

Susan Curtis — *Homeopathic Alternatives to Immunisation* Winter Press, 1994

Miranda Castro — *Homeopathy for Pregnancy, Birth and Your Baby's First Year* St. Martin's Press, 1993

Gabrielle Pinto and Murray Feldman — *Homeopathy for Children: A Parent's Guide to the Treatment of Common Childhood Illnesses* C. W. Daniels, 2000

Henrietta Wells — *Homeopathy for Children: The Practical Family Guide* Element Books, 1994

Index

• • • • •